1

Love

and

Fear

stories from
a hospice chaplain

Renshin Bunce

Gratitude

To Zenkei Blanche Hartman, who ordained me
To Myogen Steve Stücky, who taught me
To Zoketsu Norman Fischer, who caught me
when I was falling

To the Vow that carries me

and

To all of my patients and family members,
remembered or forgotten

and

To my many friends who
told me to
write

Table of Contents

Introduction

I say now that my mother was my first hospice patient. She was 77, she had cancer, and she died screaming. I can draw a line from that nightmare to my first day as a hospice chaplain, so I say now that her bad death was the last gift she gave me. That story is one of many I want to tell you. But first, let me tell you who I am.

Let's begin with this: I'm not an angel. When I say "Zen priest" and "chaplain," some people sit up a little straighter and feel they have to explain why they haven't been to church lately or apologize if they swear. Please. I'm a product of the San Francisco art world in the psychedelic 60's and a recovering alcoholic/addict whose motto was "I'll try anything twice," so I'm pretty much unshockable.

I inherited my alcoholism from my parents. My mom was an ambitious girl who moved from Murray, Utah to San Francisco to find her fortune. She was smart, tall, and beautiful, with a tremendous sense of humor, and she struck gold when she met my father, a society boy from New York. They were married in Grace Cathedral, and she joined the Junior League. But she didn't get the life she wanted. My father became a violent drunk, and she packed up my older sister and me and left him in the late 1940s when this was still a radical act. My dad sobered up and quickly met a woman who he married and stayed with for 50 years. My mom didn't remarry, and she worked as a secretary for the rest of her life. She was angry, and she drank.

I ignored her experience and advice and started my life with just one plan: to find a man, get married, and live happily ever after. I was typical of the girls of my time in that. But then, when I finally found my tribe at the art school, there was a twist in the plot. My friends and I were early adopters of psychedelic drugs, and those explorations of reality changed everything. I became more interested in creativity and freedom than in commitment and conformity, and the white picket fence didn't look so good any more as I whole-heartedly joined my generation's plunge into sex, drugs and rock and roll. I still wanted to find a man who would take care of me, but now he had to wear a black leather jacket and show his work at a good gallery.

I bounced between San Francisco, New York, and Berkeley. I typed. I modeled. I lived with a painter who stayed home all day smoking dope while I trotted off to temp jobs on Wall Street. I read about Women's Liberation in *The Village Voice* and thought maybe I should get serious about my life but I didn't know how. I was one of the pretty girls who lived in the Chelsea Hotel and waited tables at Max's Kansas City. I lived with a Madison Avenue art director who tried to commit suicide one horrible night and never finished the film I'd starred in. Big eyes and long legs got me into interesting situations, but I was still lonely and scared a lot of the time. I was one of the drug-addled salespeople at *Rolling Stone* in its early days in San Francisco. I lived with a wine importer who introduced me to a life of glamour and good food until he ran off with one of the cooks at Chez Panisse. I got pregnant and the father said he'd leave me if I didn't have an abortion, and I was so afraid of losing him that I did. I worked for Francis Coppola for a while, first at a magazine he started and then, when that failed, I put together a restaurant for his building in North Beach. I got fired a lot, and attitude was often mentioned. Boyfriends left me or I left them, and women friends were hard to find. I didn't know how to be kind. I was curious about developing an inner life and I read the *I Ching* and drew astrology charts. I carried a book by Krishnamurti around with me, but I don't think I ever read it. Nothing was ever enough.

My mother was the only friend I had left when I crashed into AA at the age of 35. I'd lost my home and my job and was drinking in North Beach and sleeping on her couch. I reached out to a clinic shrink who suggested my drinking was the problem, not the solution. My mother asked me what it was with this self-improvement project, but she loaned me the money to move into a hotel and begin to learn to live without drugs and alcohol. After my first AA meeting, I never drank or used again.

I was ten years sober when Mom called to ask me to go with her to see a doctor. He examined her and said the tumor in her stomach would kill her. Mom had always argued against treatment for others when they were dying. "Pull the plug" she'd mutter, and laugh. Now that it was her turn, though, she changed her mind. She demanded chemotherapy, and fought death with all her might.

She was in and out of the hospital for months, and I went with her to doctor's appointments or, when there was a crisis, to the emergency room. The only other person she could call was her sister, but Aunt Betty was also an alcoholic and she couldn't be counted on. My sister hadn't spoken to either of our parents for decades, so she was out. I was willing, and I was available: I was selling real estate and, although no sales meant no income, I was able to stop working to be with my mom full time. I slept by her side in the hospital, and, when they sent her home on a stretcher to die, I picked up my cat from my little studio apartment and we moved in with her.

I took care of my mom from Halloween until the end of February. A hospice nurse came once or twice a week, and left me a number to call when I had a question or needed help. I learned to give my mother a bed bath and change her diapers. I gave her morphine from a big glass bottle when she moaned. I don't remember meeting a social worker, a chaplain, or a home health aide. I felt very alone. My sister returned and sat sobbing at the bedside. My mom and Aunt Betty were thrilled she'd come back, but I thought to myself that I'd never left.

Late one night my mother started making a gurgling sound, and I phoned hospice for help. The nurse who came the next day said I was hearing the death rattle. I phoned my aunt and my sister, and they came and then, when I realized they were leaving me alone with a dying woman, I called a friend who brought dinner and stayed with me. We were talking in the living room when we heard my mother scream "NO NO NO." I ran down the hall to comfort her, and, after she quieted, was so exhausted that I fell asleep by her side. When I woke, she had stopped breathing.

When death came for my mother, it came as a stranger, and it brought terror with it. I thought then that if I had a chance to become familiar with death, it might be helpful when it came for me, as it surely would.

I went back to selling real estate. I'd been trying to parlay a used Mercedes and a wallet full of charge cards into a facade that would keep me in the game, but eventually the struggle and the mask became too painful. After 17 years, I knew I needed something else. I'd gone to the Buddhists to learn how to meditate, hoping to quiet my restless mind, and the Buddha's teachings that were woven into the meditation instruction felt like the answer to a question I hadn't known how to ask. Eventually, a dozen years of going on retreats and finding a teacher I could trust tipped the scales away from chasing men and money and toward what it felt like to sit in black robes in a silent Zendo, smelling the incense and listening to the sound of the bell.

Ten years after my mother died, although it terrified me to do it, I quit my job, cashed out my IRA to pay off my credit card debt, gave my cat away, put my books and furniture in storage, and moved to a Zen monastery. I thought moving into Zen Center, taking vows and following directions, would provide me with the family I yearned for, with a place to live and something meaningful to do for the rest of my life.

"Living in a monastery" sounds so peaceful, but, in fact, that peace is arrived at by a lot of hard work, both physical and emotional. We had no heat or electricity. The wakeup bell rang at 3:45 and we stayed busy until lights out at 9:30. We didn't choose who we bumped up against a thousand times a day, and I'm sure some of the other 50 residents were as irritated by me as I was by them. It was a hard way to live, but this centuries-old method for taming the mind works. When all of the choices I spent my energy on were removed, there was nothing left to do during long days of meditation but witness the stream of thoughts that had been running my life and, finally, find a way out of the traps I'd set for myself. I ordained as a priest, took the Japanese name my teacher gave me, and was sure I'd made the right choice. Years passed. It wasn't the safe life I'd hoped for, but I could feel it changing me, feel my swings between anxiety and depression lessen, feel a movement away from isolation and into connection.

But Zen Center doesn't want to be an old folks home, and after seven years it became clear I wasn't one of the very few people who would be allowed to live there forever. My teacher had just been named Abbot and I could have asked him to get special treatment for me, but I didn't. I was ready for some comfort. I wanted my privacy back. I wanted to eat a hamburger and get some sleep. I wanted to get my furniture out of storage and lie on my couch and read a novel.

Once again I was faced with the question of how to support myself, and now I was 65 and I was broke. I needed a new plan that included taking my vow as a priest — the vow that literally said I would save all beings, and practically meant that I would try to be helpful -- into the world. There was room for comfort in my new life, but serving others, not pleasing myself, would be the point to it.

And that's how, after 35 years of drinking heavily and looking for someone to fix me, 17 years of passing for sane in a realtor's black suit and long red fingernails, and seven years as a Zen monk, I entered a chaplaincy training program in a hospital.

When one of my chaplaincy teachers told me that most of the work for chaplains is in hospice, I thought that would be all right. It was 20 years after my mother's bad death, and I thought if I could be a hospice chaplain, I could live my vow and learn about death too. And so I have.

Now, before we get to the stories, I want to say something about patient privacy. There's a law called HIPAA (Health Insurance Portability and Accountability Act) which means I can't tell you anything that would make a patient identifiable, so I've kept details vague. In a few cases difficulties were kept from family members, and I've softened the edges of those stories to protect them. Most of the stories are a straight-out telling of what happened, as best as I can remember it. I hope you benefit from them as much as I have.

Starting Out

While I was still on staff at Zen Center, I enrolled in a year-long class at a local Buddhist center to learn how to be a chaplain. We went to monthly meetings where people talked about the work, and we were required to put in volunteer hours with actual sick people. I did mine in the local safety net hospital. A group of us were getting an orientation tour of that huge and rundown place with its one staff chaplain when a man in a black leather jacket who was leaning in the doorway of the AIDS ward said, softly, "Please come and help us" as we passed down the hall. I did.

For my first day there, I printed out a copy of the 23rd Psalm and put it in the back pocket of my new black jeans. I was so naïve that I thought I'd be visiting people in private rooms with clean sheets and curtains billowing in the breeze, and expected them to want to hear a Christian prayer. What I entered was quite the opposite, a large open ward with beds close together and light filtered through dirty windows. The staffers greeted me, but no one had the time to talk. They assumed I knew what I was doing. I made my way through the room, stopping to greet guys who were lying on their beds, talking, reading, or looking at little TVs. When I called myself a chaplain, some responded eagerly and others turned away in silence. I found a patio outside where the residents sat to smoke, and it was easier for me to sit there too and get to know some of them. I saw the way they took care of each other, the ones who still had some energy watching over those whose disease had progressed. One day one of the residents was dying and they asked me to sit with him inside the curtains that were drawn around his bed, and so I held someone's hand in his final hours for the first time on that charity ward. Another resident asked to speak to me privately, and so on a wood-en bench in a hall of a city hospital I heard my first confession. Through those months, I knew so little of what I was seeing that I made a lot of mistakes. Those AIDS patients were forgiving; they began to show me what a chaplain can do, and the possibilities for connection created by that role.

After that, I was convinced I wanted to work as a professional chaplain, so I applied to a number of programs in Clinical Pastoral Education (CPE), the year-long residency most employers require. I was thrilled when a local hospital accepted me, and surprised when one of my teachers asked if I could afford it – I'd been living below the poverty level at Zen Center for so long, I thought $2,000 a month was big money. I kept living in the temple, and nearly half of the stipend went to my room and board. For the familiarity of the meditation hall in the morning and the comfort of the dining room at night, it was a bargain. I pulled black blouses and skirts out of my storage unit so I'd look the part, and felt the whole world open in front of me the first time I walked out of the front door and into my new life.

I was joined with four other CPE students, all of them a generation younger than I, all of them Christians fulfilling a requirement for the seminaries they were attending. We met in a windowless basement room and listened as our supervisor lectured us about hand-washing and patient privacy and gave us his views on spiritual care. Finally we got to see patients. I was full of uncertainty. My sales experience helped me get into the room, but then I didn't know what to do. I didn't want to look foolish, didn't want to bother anyone, and I didn't want to be rejected. I only wanted to offer superb advice and heal everyone I met.

I made a lot of mistakes because I was trying to look like I knew more than I did. I talked too much. I thought people expected a chaplain to be a Christian, and so I prayed and talked about God. A lot. I realized that, instead of being who I was, I was being who I thought someone else wanted me to be. When I finally relaxed and started listening, I could let my patients teach me how to be a chaplain. Then, through trial and error, leaving a visit and realizing I'd acted like an idiot, or feeling during a conversation that something real was happening, I found a way to be who I am without making the visit be about me, and to find out what will make the patient feel seen and heard and safe.

Finally, though, most of my education took place when I was on call at night, when the small number of regular professional chaplains who knew what they were doing were home asleep in their warm beds and my beeper went off to call me to the hospital for an emergency. In those cases the learning curve was dizzyingly steep.

The first time I was called to an emergency in the ICU, it was at the end of a routine day, just when I was looking forward to going home. A young husband and father had died suddenly, and his mother was in one of the family rooms outside of the unit. She was screaming. Other relatives milled around, but the chairs on either side of her were vacant. I sat next to her, put my arm around her, and handed her Kleenex. She calmed down, smiled, and thanked me.

I asked whether she had seen the body and, since she hadn't, walked her and her other two sons into the ICU so they could say goodbye. The dead man had suddenly dropped to the ground at his construction job and attempts to resuscitate him had brought him here. The doctor said a weakness in his heart had killed him. His body waited in the ICU as the bureaucracy moved him and his family through the system. I hoped that seeing his body, his young handsome face with no spark of life left in it, might help his mother understand what had happened, to absorb his death, so she could begin to grieve his loss. When she stood by his side, she simply looked at him and wept. Her other two sons, pink with life, stood with her and they cried too.

When we went back to the waiting area, I felt relieved – I'd survived the on call and I'd been helpful. I found the dead man's young wife downstairs in the chapel with a friend, frantic on her cellphone as she made call after call to report the tragedy. I asked if she wanted to see her husband's body and she waved me away and turned back to her phone. Her friend mouthed a thank you and I left.

The whole thing had taken about an hour and I was able to get home in time for dinner. Later, in the comfort of my own room, I realized I had been treating this tragedy like a task, but it was much larger than that. I put my work clothes back on and drove to the ICU. The patient's body had been taken to the morgue and most of the family had left, yet the mother was still in the room where we'd first met, and she was screaming again, refusing to leave. There was nothing to say but I did find the courage to sit with her through the night. It was only when someone arrived to take her home that I knew my job, which was to bear witness to her sorrow, was finished.

Some weeks later, when I was still very new on the job, my beeper woke me from my sleep, and when I dialed the number it showed, the operator said I was needed in the ICU. I dressed, hurried through the silent halls of Zen Center, and drove across town to the hospital.

As I entered the unit, before I could find a nurse to ask what the crisis was, a woman rushed up. She saw my short hair, sensible shoes, and black blouse and skirt, and asked if I was a nun. Surprised, I nodded and mumbled something about being a priest. She was satisfied. She said her brother -in-law was dying and her sister needed help. She walked me to them and left.

Inside the small ICU cubicle, I saw a man in bed, one of his legs in a complicated metal cage on top of the sheets, and a young woman clinging to him, crying. He was calling out in pain and she was begging him not to die. She looked up at me and, after I said I was the chaplain, shook her head and said she wasn't religious. I said her sister had asked me to come and say a prayer. She stared at me and then nodded. I walked to the other side of the bed and opened my Gideon Bible to read the 23rd Psalm.

The patient was a big man who appeared to be in his fifties. When he turned his head in my direction, I saw his face was twisted in pain and the whites of his eyes were red with blood. I tried not to flinch. He turned back to his wife. I fumbled my way through the psalm, wanting to help without interfering, and then stepped back. I knew I couldn't show up, say a prayer that neither of them believed in, and leave; but I didn't know what else I was supposed to do.

There was no room in the cubicle, so I sat on a chair in the corridor, just outside the open doorway, trying to be there without being in the way. The noises from other rooms, patients moaning and machines beeping, spoke of the suffering that surrounded me. Nurses hurried back and forth. I closed my eyes. I chanted silently to myself, calling on Quan Yin, the goddess of compassion. For the first time since my beeper went off, my heart stopped racing. I became calm.

And then it came to me: I was a visual reminder of the great fact that what was happening here was more than a physical event. My sitting there with my nun's hair and my black clothes told everyone who saw me, both patients and staff, that there is a spiritual dimension to this business of living and dying. That's what I was there for, not for any wise words I could say or magic I could perform. No one could stop the patient from dying and breaking his wife's heart, but possibly I could help them remember that this body is not the whole story about who we are.

When I left, one of the nurses told me the patient had shattered his leg in a car crash many months earlier and had been living on painkillers until, finally, they'd destroyed his organs. He was bleeding internally and that's why his eyes were bright red. She smiled as if to acknowledge we were on the same team, two professionals who knew that there are times when the release of death is not the worst thing that can happen.

Though I was stunned by the whole thing -- a rookie in way over her head -- the understanding that came to me as

I sat in that corridor has stayed with me through the years: the chaplain's presence can remind everyone that life and death are more than a physical event.

One of my worst on calls in the hospital was for a young Mexican woman whose baby had been a stillbirth. I don't know whether prenatal care would have made a difference for her baby, but the first thing the maternity ward nurses said when I arrived was that she hadn't seen a doc-tor because she couldn't afford it. It was after midnight and they were tired and sad and eager to hand over the bur-den of this death to someone else. That's why they, not the patient's family, had called for a chaplain. They'd also called for a Catholic priest, and he had already come and gone.

One looked up from her paperwork and told me, "They're in one of the birthing rooms. The mother and her husband came in earlier today because she was in pain. She was about six months pregnant – they aren't sure. A lot of family have shown up but no one speaks much English. Remember to ask if they want to have a picture taken with the baby before we take away the remains. Thank you for coming."

Walking the long hall, I saw about a dozen men in work clothes, some whispering to each other, most standing silently, some praying, working the rosary beads they held. In the room I saw more men standing, and a young woman in the bed. The dimly-lit space was painted a soft mint green, the bed arranged in an archway so it looked like a throne. The birthing room had been designed for joy, for new life, not for this.

I saw a portable bassinet in the middle of the room and realized the baby's corpse was there. I stepped to its side and looked down to see the tiny body wrapped in a too-large receiving blanket, its face uncovered, its eyelids still sealed shut. Out of instinct, needing to do something, I reached down and put my hand on the corpse and said, "Oh beautiful baby." It was as if I'd flipped a switch.

The people in the room came to life. One man walked to the other side of the bassinet and stared at the baby. I assumed he was the father. He was wearing jeans and a dusty blue chambray shirt -- he must have been working outdoors when he got the call to take his wife to the hospital. His eyes met mine. I gestured to the body. He lifted it and started to cry. He walked back to the other men and they looked at the baby, took it, passed it around, weeping over it, loving it.

Finally, he carried the baby to the bed and sat by his wife's side. Together, they held the body and cried.

I stepped to them, said "Sorry." I don't speak Spanish and using the translation line on the phone seemed intrusive, even unnecessary. I made a picture-taking gesture, motioned toward the three of them, asked with my eyes whether they wanted this. They nodded.

"Gracias," she said.

I stepped back to the wall. I watched. The room was full of life and death and sorrow. When I went back down the hall, past the silent standing men who didn't yet know the whole horrible day was about to come to an end, I told the nurse I thought the family was ready to have the memory picture taken.

In the years since that case in which, in a move of instinct born from desperation, I showed that family how to approach their grief, I've entered many rooms where old people lie dead and their middle-aged children sit around them, waiting for someone to tell them what to do. I always touch the corpse and, if it's been a peaceful death, say how beautiful they look. I learned how to do that with this family.

When I finished my formal training in the hospital, I had a terrible time finding a job. It was 2008, the world economy had crashed, and no one was hiring. I had left the safety of Zen Center to do a final three month unit of CPE in a hospital across the bay, and was living in a dark little apartment far from the companionship of temple life. I fought off depression as I filed online job applications and heard nothing in return.

Finally, to my joy and surprise, I got a two month temp job as a hospice chaplain in Oregon, covering for someone who was out on sick leave. The kind woman who conducted the interview over Skype asked whether I thought I might be lonely. "No!" I cried. "I'm very self-sufficient!" I hadn't done home visits before and I'd never lived in Portland, but I gave away my goldfish, packed my old car, and drove for ten hours to an apartment I found on Craigslist.

After I shadowed the other chaplains and learned the electronic charting system, I was pretty much on my own. I just had to figure out who needed a visit, where they lived, who else I could see in the same general area, and then get in my car and go.

My days felt similar to going from bed to bed in the hospital, but on a much larger scale as I set my radio on NPR and drove around the Oregon countryside. The other chaplains were busy seeing their own patients and I didn't get to know any of the nurses. I had overestimated myself: I was lonely. I missed the fellowship I had felt strolling the halls of the hospital, and the urgency of being called to the ICU. I had many visits where both the patient and I seemed to wonder what I was doing there as we chatted politely.

And yet, I found I liked home care. I liked having time alone between patients to think about them, and the freedom to maybe even stop and have a cup of coffee and sit in the sun and read the paper. I also came to appreciate visiting people in their own homes; I was surrounded with information as soon as I walked in the door. If there were family pictures on the wall, it was useful to ask about them. Other mementos helped, too, such as quilts and books and record collections. I learned about board and care homes, houses that looked like any other from the street and held four or five residents and a couple of caregivers. I met a lot of bed-ridden people in places like that, and began to learn that I didn't have to strive to bring a serious spiritual message: being a friendly visitor was enough. I met a woman lying in bed in a room with no radio or television, no books or magazines. I asked her what she did all day. She said, "See that tree over there?" I said yes. "I watch that tree" she said. I still find it comforting to know that watching a tree can be enough.

Once my manager stopped me as I was leaving at the end of the day and asked me to visit a woman who was dying. When I arrived at the facility, I found that there was a volunteer at her bedside. I thought I was there to say a quick deathbed prayer, but the volunteer, a man who had more experience than I, showed me something more. The patient was alone in the world, and together we cleaned her, brushed her hair and put her in a pretty nightgown so she'd be ready for what was coming. We sat with her for hours that night, keeping her company, being her family.

A month or so into that job, I met a young woman who was dying of cancer. She had gone to a place overseas that promised a cure when she was first diagnosed, but now the disease had spread and she had returned home to Oregon to use its Death with Dignity law to end her life. She told me her pain was unbearable but she hated what heavy drugs did to her, so her days and nights revolved around the search for a balance between pain control and consciousness. She said it wasn't a life worth living. When she talked about taking the lethal drugs my company's doctor would provide for her, I told her I understood. I said no one would blame her. She was interested in Buddhism, so she lay on a velvet couch in the living room with her eyes closed, and I read to her from Pema Chodron's book *When Things Fall Apart*. She was one of the few patients I felt connected to in that time.

Maybe I was like many hospice patients, nodding my head and agreeing but not really believing death was coming; when she took the lethal drugs and died just days after one of our visits, I was devastated. I thought the hospice doctor had failed, that he should have found drugs that kept her both pain free and alert; and I blamed her, and thought she should have stayed home and started treatment when she was first diagnosed instead of running off and searching for a miracle. This was the first time I felt grief for one of my patients. The other chaplains were busy with their own patients and I didn't know who else I could talk to about this young woman in particular and physician aid-in-dying in general, so I kept my confusion to myself.

I was lonely in that job in many ways. Later I would learn to speak up in weekly team meetings with nurses and social workers, but I doubt I ever said a word in those two months. Now I understand that forming relationships with co-workers is essential to doing the work -- it's just too hard to do alone -- and also that all disciplines have something useful to contribute to patient care. But back then I was too intimidated: I listened and left. I knew a few people in Portland and there were a flurry of dinners and movie dates when I first arrived, but that tapered off too. I missed the familiarity of my neighborhood, the grocery store where I could find everything I was looking for, and, most of all, my friends. When the regular chaplain returned and my assignment ended, I was ready to go home.

I returned to collecting unemployment and reading job postings online - but even with some experience to add to my resume, I didn't get any interviews. I could check the box that asked if I was ordained, and the one that asked whether I'd completed CPE, but couldn't claim I had a graduate degree in divinity.

Christians receive a Masters of Divinity (M.Div.) when they graduate from seminary. Zen Center, of course, didn't grant any degrees, and it became clear that I needed an M.Div. if I was going to get a job. There was a graduate program in Buddhist studies that was starting locally, and going there would have earned me the degree, but it would also have taken me two or three years and put me more deeply in debt. Someone told me the Association of Professional Chaplains grants an M.Div. equivalency to Buddhists, and I applied. It took me one month to put together a three inch thick document proving that seven years of

Zen training equaled 72 units (7200 hours) of graduate studies. It worked: I was offered a hospice job contingent on the degree, and the letter granting me the equivalency arrived that same week. I was finally going to get to work.

When I tell people I work in hospice, they almost always say the same thing: "That must be so hard." What I think they mean is, it must be so hard to be around death. After many years and visits, I can say that death often means release for my patients, and being a part of it is frequently a blessing.

When I agree with people who say working in hospice sounds hard, what I mean is, witnessing the suffering of others is hard. Seeing a patient in pain while nursing home staff ignore her is hard. Listening to families fight while someone lies next to them dying is hard. Visiting people for months, coming to love them, and then losing them is hard. Being powerless is hard and my work reminds me that ultimately we're all dealing with forces much greater than we are, and many times it's clear those forces are beyond human control. A small number of my patients and family members say everything is God's will, and I'm happy for them but I don't believe in that God. I believe in love and in each of us doing our best and sometimes it seems that the things I see could be better and I try to help when it's like that.

Another thing that's hard is, hospice is part of health-care, and in modern American healthcare we're all small cogs in a large corporate machine designed for profit, not for kindness and caring.

The first job I got was with a for-profit hospice that was the powerhouse provider in the area. When we met with management once a month, they cheered the billowing patient census and lectured us on entering chart notes correctly to get the maximum Medicare reimbursement for our work. At that company I couldn't find any support for the feelings I had at being so close to death, no place to tell the stories I needed to hear out loud to help me make sense of what I'd seen, or even anyone to ask for advice. I struggled. I was so naïve: the first time I had a job review with the clinical boss, I shared some of my feelings about the company with her. I thought she'd want to know. I told her it seemed we were in such a rush to make money that we'd forgotten our primary function was to offer comfort and caring.

She looked at me in astonishment and barked "If you feel that way, why do you keep working here?" Good question, and saying it was the only offer I got after a long job hunt wasn't the right answer.

"Because you hold the keys to the kingdom: you give me access to people who are dying" was what I said, and that was true too.

At that company, I learned that, since hospice is a Medicare benefit, Medicare writes the rules. Being on hospice means all treatment is for comfort and not for cure. It means no more trips to the hospital for infections or falls unless there's something as serious as a broken bone – we come to the patient when there's a problem. A patient becomes hospice-eligible when a doctor certifies they have a terminal illness and appear to have less than six months to live. This doesn't mean they're going to die in six months or that we stop visiting if they don't, but they do have to show decline to stay on service. We go through rigorous reviews every few months to make sure that they're still hospice-eligible, and if they're stable, we have to discharge them or Medicare takes back the money they've paid for their care and this can be disastrous to a small local hospice.

Medicare requires that new admissions be seen by each team member within five days. After that first contact, I decide how often to visit. I look for the people who are lonely, who are worried or afraid, or those who simply appreciate a little variety in their routine. I've learned to keep an eye out for the family members doing the grindingly hard work of caregiving, and visit them too. If I don't think I can do any good, I don't visit, and there are people who refuse to even meet me. Some people are in between, neither eager nor dismissive, and I visit them in the hope of establishing a connection so I can be available if the time comes that they need someone to talk to.

I respond when my nurses ask me to make a visit, whether I think it will help the patient or not. I want my co-workers to know I'm on their side, and to feel that the patient's emotional/spiritual needs are being met and they don't have to be the ones doing it.

Although hospice is designed to allow people to stay out of the hospital when they're dying, the system seems to assume there's someone at home who can care for them, who has the physical strength and skill to administer drugs, prepare food, change diapers, and keep the patient from falling or wandering out the front door. When there's no one who can do this, unless the patient or their family can afford to pay live-in caregivers, the patient's home will be in a facility. Medicare doesn't pay room and board, and Medicare doesn't send anyone to help people at home. In California, that's where Medicaid, known here as Medi-Cal, comes in, either providing caregivers for a maximum of four hours a day, or paying for a bed in a nursing home.

I visit people in their own homes, alone or with family members or paid caregivers; in group homes where six or so old folks sit around a television all day, supervised by one or two caregivers who vary vastly in how much they care about the residents; in large senior living facilities where people move from independent living to assisted living while their monthly payments rise accordingly; and in skilled nursing facilities, which, again unless the patient is wealthy, are the sort of understaffed and impersonal institutional setting that most of us think of when we hear "nursing home." There are a few free-standing residential hospices for people in the final weeks of life, and I visit people there, too.

People often call hospice workers angels and tell me I have a calling to do this work. That may be true, but it sits side by side with the hard reality of the corporate world, and I had to adjust my idea of the way things should be if I wanted to be a part of it. I found a support group for professional caregivers and it's probably because of that wonderful group of doctors, nurses, therapists and chaplains that I have been able to stay in the work long enough to learn a way to tolerate its difficulties without closing my heart.

So I hope that's enough about the business of hospice, enough about the fussing around with money and paperwork, with satisfying the government and pleasing my bosses. Because finally, when all of that is taken care of, what's left is the visit.

In ten years, I've never stopped asking: What is it to be a chaplain? What is the chaplain supposed to do? What does it mean to help?

Being a Zen priest brought me to this work, but I don't do it as "a Buddhist chaplain." It's my job to serve everyone. I come along, a tall woman on the older side of middle age with short brown hair and a pleasant face, usually wearing a black skirt and a white blouse, and I sit down, look my patient in the eyes, and we talk.

A friend recently questioned whether all of my well-intentioned words make any difference when the chips are down. He said, "The question is whether she will be able to remember what you said when she needs to, even if she agrees with it whole-heartedly. This is death. Very few people are wired to do that well."

There was a time in my training when I felt the futility of it. I know how slow change is, how we can hear wise words over and over until the time comes that we understand them, and even then it might be longer still before we can act on them. Still, I have to try. I talk. I take everything I know and distill it down and hope when the time comes, those words will be something they can use, something that will make a difference. I think of all the times in my life when I would have really appreciated some guidance, and I keep talking. Or I listen. Or I just sit. There's no formula for what happens next – that's the point, and that's the challenge.

Finding Connection

To be a chaplain isn't to be the person with all the answers. It's just the opposite. It's to meet strangers who are reeling from hearing the word *hospice*, remain open to their pain, and try to figure out what we can do to help. Our patients, family members, and even longtime paid caregivers find themselves in a place where they never wanted to be. They need a guide, and hospice workers are the ones who are familiar with the territory. Many need to hear about the process, need help in identifying the unfamiliar feelings they're having as they lose control over their lives. I'm a big talker, an explainer, a normalizer, and that role is comfortable for me. Then there are people who are lonely and want some company and aren't so interested in talking about death or meaning, and I need to be there for them too.

Finally, we have many patients whose minds are affected by their disease – maybe through dementia, or maybe because they're on heavy pain control drugs, and I visit them too, often to simply sit and be there, another human being by their side. It's these visits with people who are no longer able to talk, to reason, to ask questions, to argue, that force me once again to ask myself what help is.

There is one case that I continue to turn to for guidance. Since the patient's diagnosis was dementia, I expected him to be an old man – but the person I found sitting in a wheelchair in a facility dining room was in his early fifties. He was dressed in dad clothes, a nice plaid shirt and khaki pants, and he was younger than anyone else in the room, including me. The contrast between his youthful face and his damaged brain was painful to witness.

I learned that his wife had put him in this facility and left town. I felt sorry for him, so, whenever I was in the area, I made sure we spent a few minutes together. Sometimes his gaze was dull and unfocused, and sometimes, briefly, his eyes met mine and he struggled to hold contact.

His wife returned after a few weeks, and we had a care conference with her and several staff members. She was dressed crisply in slacks and a tucked-in shirt, and she seemed nervous, but people often are at the start of one of these things. Before we began, she dialed her daughter on her cell phone, put it on speaker, and set it on a table in the middle of the group. While the phone was ringing, she turned to me to say that she was a volunteer chaplain herself. I smiled and said that was great, and she said "Yes, we're Evangelical Christians and I bring the good news to people." Her daughter answered and the meeting began before we could say more. My experience is that Evangelicals don't welcome Buddhists and I was glad for the interruption.

We reviewed the patient's history, and she told us that the first signs of dementia had appeared about five years earlier as the kind of ordinary forgetfulness, the lost words and misplaced objects, that middle-aged people joke about. But his memory had deteriorated so rapidly that within a year he could no longer work, and she had taken early retirement to care for him at home. Finally, when he was in diapers and unable to walk or talk, her daughter had convinced her to put him in this facility. Then she'd found tenants for their house and put their furniture in storage, and now she was driving around the country, visiting family and friends, living nowhere and trying to follow her daughter's advice to start a new life for herself.

The team members introduced ourselves, raising our voices so the daughter could hear. When I said I was the chaplain, her daughter's voice called out from the cellphone speaker, "Do you accept Christ as your savior?"

I tried to sidestep the question because I had become attached to the patient, and I wanted to keep visiting him. I told her that, as a hospice chaplain, all of the work I do is nondenominational, and that I'm more concerned with meeting the needs of the patient than with my own beliefs.

With her, my sidestep didn't work. The tinny voice on the speakerphone asked, "If you don't accept Christ as your Savior, then what are you?" When I said I was a Zen Buddhist priest, there was a pause, and then she asked, "Don't you have Christian chaplains?" She sounded plaintive. Her mother remained silent.

Ordinarily I'd say yes and tell the family that I could arrange for someone else to visit. But in this case, I thought the patient was lonely, and I thought I was being helpful. I said that we did have Christian chaplains but, because all of us worked in our own geographic territories, he'd get more attention if the family would let me keep visiting. I assured her I could honor the family's beliefs when I met with her father. We moved on; the issue was left unresolved.

He declined rapidly. Soon he could no longer sit upright and I found him slumped forward in the wheel-chair, unable to raise his head and meet my eyes. Eventually the care home staff stopped getting him out of bed. When I visited, I sat with him, greeted him, chattered, and then remained silent. I always said a prayer before I left, putting my hand on his head and praying to God to bring him peace, to help him know he was safe, to help him know he was loved.

This went on for months. I usually called the patient's wife and left a message after my visit. Sometimes she called back from wherever she was, and some of these conversations were long and friendly. She seemed to be lonely too. Sometimes she told me she'd been in town and seen him, and we talked about the difficulty of watching him slip away. I told her about something called "anticipatory grief" — the sorrow we feel when the person we love is gone but the body continues to live. She said that sounded right to her.

One day when I arrived I found him lying, clothed, on his bed. I pulled up a chair and sat next to him, leaning against the bed rails. His roommate often sat across the room in a reclining chair, mumbling and groaning, but on this day we were alone. I offered my usual greeting; then, since this was a rare day when his gaze met mine directly, I wondered aloud if there was anything I could do for him, if there was anything I could do to help. He lifted his hand and moved it toward me slowly. I watched. His finger came to rest on the button of my shirt. He plucked at it. "What?" I asked, and he pulled more urgently. I think that he was asking me to undo that button. I smiled and told him I couldn't do that. I leaned back in my chair and he slowly put his hand back on the bed.

A satellite radio tuned to modern Christian music appeared on his bedside table. One day I turned the dial until I found an oldies station, and I sang along to Elvis Presley and the Beatles while he lay listening. I should have turned the dial back when I left, but I didn't. On my next visit there was a big sign saying not to touch the radio.

Then my manager said the patient's daughter had phoned and demanded that the company provide a Christian chaplain. I don't know why she made that call after all those months and wondered if it was because I'd messed with that silly radio, but I was really upset. I wanted to keep visiting him. After I calmed down, I phoned her mother and asked if I could continue if we added a Christian chaplain's visits to mine. She was still the legal decision maker, and she agreed. In that conversation, she told me that her daughter had been the one who had "urged her to get on with her life," and that the girl had told her that "he was so demented that he didn't know the difference." And that's what she was trying to do: get on with her life. If she had asked my opinion, I would have argued against her daugh-ter's view, but she didn't, and I remained silent.

I think this is the only time I haven't simply followed a family member's request. I'm glad I didn't, for the patient's sake and for mine.

One day, I sat by his side with my hand on his arm while he lay on the bed, unable to respond as I called him by name and reminded him who I was; I told him the date and commented on the time of year. Then I was quiet. On this day the radio was off; there was no roommate, no noise, no activity, nothing. Just his arm and my hand.

I thought about what I was doing.

When I met him, I had seen his isolation, and I had wanted to reassure him that he wasn't alone even though his family had left him with strangers. But now that felt arrogant; it was too much about me, and it was presumptuous to think I could take the place of his family.

I sat and waited. I watched the late winter light move across the room. I had an image of a reservoir inside me that was filled by the hours I'd spent in meditation; it was as if I was siphoning off peace from the reservoir and sharing it with him. That was nice, and it may have even been true, but it still wasn't the whole thing. I sat some more.

I wondered whether my task might be to let him know that he was still seen and still a part of the human race, no matter what his circumstances. And then it became clear that my visit was about connection — a connection that was much larger than two people, much larger than any words I could say, a connection that could only be realized, not created. And it didn't go from me to him, it arose between the two of us equally. So I held on to his arm to let him know, not that I was there, or that he was, but that we were. I wasn't there to prevent loneliness, I was there to remind him, and myself, that we are never alone. That we are all connected, always, whether there is another person sitting by our side or not. There are many words for this and one of them is God. Another is love.

In the years since that day, I have been at many similar bedsides, and I think *connection* as I sit next to a person who is still very much alive, even though they can no longer remember who or where they are.

Years after I sat with that young man with dementia, I was assigned another young man to care for. He had a brain tumor and, although he was intelligent and successful, when we met he couldn't remember where he was or why he was there, so he lived in a state of confusion. He wasn't unhappy, just bewildered.

He could no longer walk, and his speech was limited to short sentences, but he wasn't just propped up in front of a television set, as so many patients are. A nephew had stepped in to manage his care, and hired private caregivers who would roll him around the perimeter of the care facility to let him feel the sun on his skin. They helped him to eat in the dining room. They made sure he attended the facility's group activities — I sat to the side and watched as this brilliant man proudly called out the answers to the simple questions that appeared on a screen in a room full of nodding old people.

When we were together, I chattered about the weather, the world, the care he was getting. I asked whether he understood what was going on with him, and he'd say "No" or "Can't understand." I'd tell him that he was sick and that he needed people to take care of him and keep him safe. I believe life and death are easier for most of us when we understand what's going on. In that moment, at least, he understood.

He got worse gradually. He could no longer sit in the wheelchair. He became bedbound, diapered, and was eating less and sleeping more. Now that he needed more care, his nephew moved him to a special hospice house where a fleet of women in pastel-colored scrubs drifted in and out of his room throughout the day and a nurse was always present.

When I visited him there, I found him awake and alone. The television was turned to one of those morning talk shows, with three women sitting around a table and blabbing about a movie star.

"That's ridiculous," I said. "Do you want to watch that?" He shook his head "No" with as much vigor as he could summon. I turned the sound off and began to fuss around the room, tidying things up, looking for something better on the TV, trying to turn on the music on his phone. I gave him a drink of water from the glass on the bedside table. Finally, I sat down.

"Talk," he said.

"You want me to talk?" I asked.

He nodded. "Can't understand," he said.

"Do you mean you can't understand where you are? You can't understand what's happening?" He nodded again.

"You're in a safe place because you're sick and you need care. Your room is pretty, isn't it?" He nodded again.

Then I asked, "Do you remember what's been happening to you in these last months?" He shook his head.

"Can't understand. Can't understand."

"You have a tumor in your brain. It's growing, and that's why you're getting weaker. That's why you need this care. This place where you're living is intended for people who are near the end of life. That's true for you. It's very sad. We don't know how much time you have left but death is drawing near."

"Oh my gosh," he said. "Really, I didn't know."

"But you're safe for a larger reason than the roof over your head and the kind people who are caring for you. We are safe because we are always a part of the large web of connection. You and I were connected before we met, and we are even more firmly connected now. This is the safety we yearn for. And connection is not limited to people. You're connected to the wisteria vine on the fence, the mountains in the distance, the stars in the sky. We are not alone." He was nodding, almost smiling.

"We use the image of Indra's net," here I raised my hands to hold the fingers on my right hand horizontally and those on the left vertically. "Each person is a jewel in the net. Each time the net is plucked, the whole thing moves. When one person is touched, we all feel it. We can't see these connections, but they are always there. We call them love. We call them God."

"Yes," he repeated. "Yes."

I'd been by the side of the bed in a straight-backed chair, sitting still to concentrate while I talked. I reached forward and stroked his arm, from the elbow to his hand. He closed his eyes and gasped with pleasure. I continued to touch his arm and then rubbed the top of his head. Then his look of surprise faded and he was calm again. He went back to sleep.

Another time I arrived and again the caregivers had left his television tuned to the daytime shows they preferred. Ads went by on the screen. Finally I said, "Wow, that's a lot of ads." He replied: "It doesn't matter. It doesn't matter." Still I kept turning the television off, fussing, fiddling with his phone so it would stream Mozart through a speaker. I do this because it's what I would want if I were lying helpless in bed.

Eventually he lost speech, even the one or two words, but his eyes still met mine. He lay in his bed, slowly moving his legs and arms, looking at me or at the trees outside, waiting for his life to end. I read to him or just sat quietly.

A year after his symptoms first appeared, he lay in a hospital bed with his eyes closed, his cheeks sunken and his color pale. A meal was a syringe of Ensure put in his mouth by a nurse, and a concentrator pumped oxygen into his lungs through a nasal cannula. His nephew and I sat by his side and talked that day, aware, even hoping, that he could hear us. The nephew told me about the family, about the pride the patient's parents felt in his accomplishments. I described the balance between fighting and acceptance that is every patient's challenge, and said that it appeared that he no longer had any life left to fight for, that death was coming and it was time for surrender.

I think he heard me. He died peacefully two days later. I'm still linked to him.

Another patient I experienced connection with was a young woman with cancer who was at home with a private caregiver. Caregivers can be territorial, and they can make it hard for me to get to the patient because they think they know better. That's how it was in this case — the caregiver brushed me off so many times when I called to visit that I gave up. Finally our nurse asked me to try again: she said the patient was failing and she was asking what dying was like. I called and got to see her.

The apartment she was living in wasn't fancy, but it was exquisite. Every thing in it had clearly been carefully chosen and precisely placed. The patient was a small figure in a huge bed with puffy white linens and, of all things, stuffed toys. She was beautiful. She was also very sick. This was her second cancer. She'd knocked the first one out several yeas ago with chemo and radiation, but treatment hadn't slowed this one down.

In our first visit we talked about jewelry and clothes. She told me she was a writer. She'd crossed the country because of a man and ended up on her own. She had a grown son and they were close. I asked, finally, when we'd been talking long enough that I thought she could trust me but not so long that she was exhausted, about fear. Was she afraid of what was happening? "I'm okay" was all she said. I told her I'd come back the next week and she agreed.

But next week the paid caregiver answered the phone and said the patient was too tired for visitors. I called every week for a while and then gave up after my visits were refused. And then, again, the nurse asked me to see her. She said the patient was dying. She was frightened and she wanted to talk about it. When I phoned, I told the paid caregiver that the patient had been asking for me and I made it past her.

That visit was different. That was the visit where I talked about death as a natural process, about how good we are at pain control, how many people loved her.

She smiled.

"You are loved. And you are safe."

"Yes."

Then again I'd call and the caregiver would tell me not to visit, saying the patient was tired or asleep. In our weekly meeting, the nurse asked how my visits were going. When I told her that I hadn't been able to get past the caregiver for another visit, the social worker laughed and told me to just go – just show up on the front porch and ring the bell. The patient would be home.

I did. The caregiver was talking on the phone when she opened the door. We nodded and she stood aside as I went back to the bedroom.

The patient was already a small woman, and now she was tiny. The cancer was eating her up. Her arms were bone thin but her stomach billowed, showing the tumor that was growing. Her eyes were huge and she was awake and smiling. I reminded her that we'd met before "and we liked each other." She agreed, maybe remembering and maybe being polite. This visit was much like the last: I reminded her that her disease was progressing and now she was taking more pain drugs, that she was loved, that we would take care of her. She paid close attention and nodded.

When I left, the caregiver held her phone away from her ear and asked me who I was. I showed her my badge and she nodded. On my next visit, the same woman opened the door. I asked how the patient was and she said "Fine. She's sleeping." I said I'd go on up and she agreed.

When I came into the room, the patient was awake. Her television was on, tuned to the station that shows "Law & Order" reruns. I greeted her and she smiled and said hello. Between the disease and the drugs, she was drifty and dreamy. This is when I hope our previous visits have laid enough of a base that she remembers me as a friend, as someone she can trust.

"Are you comfortable?" She nodded.

"Do you remember me? I'm Ren the Chaplain. You and I have had some really nice visits." She nodded again.

The paid caregiver appeared.

"Are you comfortable?" she asked.

"She is" I said, as the patient nodded.

And then the caregiver began this activity that I guessed was about proving to me that she knew what she was doing, as she began adjusting the patient, lowering the head of the bed, pulling her body up, taking pillows out here and putting them in there. I sat silently and watched. It seemed to take quite a long time.

She left.

"Is that better?" I asked.

She shook her head No and we laughed.

I reminded her again that I was the chaplain and that she and I had had visits before and again she nodded.

Suddenly she asked, "What's that?" Her voice was soft and her words were slurred, but she pointed to the foot of the bed.

"What? The bedspread?"

"That pack of cigarettes."

"Ah, I don't see any cigarettes there. Do you smoke? Do you want one?"

She shook her head no, laughed, and returned her eyes to my face. It was the morphine talking.

"How's the fear?"

"Fear" she answered. It was a statement.

"You're afraid of what's happening?"

"Afraid."

"This is just death. You're okay. I mean, I know that's easy for me to say, you're the one who's doing it, not me, but this is the very natural thing that we all know is coming. It's just coming too soon for you, but you've been getting ready for a while. What I've heard from people who are going through it is, it's such a huge change, it's going into the unknown. And you have to do it alone."

She was nodding, agreeing. She whispered "Alone."

"We're afraid because we think that we're separate and we have to keep our walls up, but there's something else going on and I think you already know about that. That you're a part of the universe and will never be separate from that no matter what happens to your body."

Her eyes were wide. "Really?"

"Yes, and you can do that yourself. You can remember that you're connected.

"And there's something else I've heard about working with the fear of death. I heard this in a talk from a great American Zen master. He said his wife was dying and that she was facing it with an attitude of curiosity, asking over and over, 'What is this?' If you're engaging with curiosity, there's no room for fear."

She was taking all of this well.

Then she asked in a whisper if I could do her a favor: "Could you just reach your hand back and get that big ball?" I reached my hand up and back extravagantly, asked "Like this?" and she nodded.

"There I am but I don't see a ball." That seemed to be okay too. She laughed again.

"You know another thing I'm seeing, you're sort of halfway there. Between the disease and the drugs, you're already in another place, aren't you?"

"Yes I guess that's what this is."

"And you're comfortable?"

"Comfortable."

"How's the fear now?"

"No fear now."

We continued sitting. I chatted a little. She pointed to the television set. One episode of "Law & Order" had concluded and the next had started. I saw a body lying in a woods and heard people saying 'rape.' I asked, "Do you know that that's a television show? Do you know that's not real?" She looked puzzled.

For the next few minutes I navigated through the unfamiliar remote control, looking for something different for her to watch. I found *The Karate Kid* and managed to change the channel. She was really happy. Then she closed her eyes. I waited. She didn't reopen them. I'd caught her window of energy and now she would sleep.

I walked downstairs. The paid caregiver was talking on her cell phone again. I smiled and said thank you when she opened the door for me to leave.

I visited twice a week until I went on vacation. When I returned in two weeks, her face had turned into a death mask, but she could still talk. I asked about the fear, and she said "No fear."

She said "Ready."

The house was freezing. The paid caregiver who was on duty that day – it was a weekend, so it wasn't the one I'd seen before - said she couldn't get the heater to work. I poked around at the wall control and then found the landlady's name on the patient's cell phone and called her for help. She said she'd get it fixed.

After the visit, I phoned her son for the first time. I introduced myself and began to talk. He interrupted. "What is the point to this call?"

"I just wanted to let you know how your mother was doing and see how you are."

"We're beginning palliative sedation tomorrow. There's nothing to talk about."

Palliative sedation is a chemical coma. We use it for patients who can't find comfort. It puts them to sleep so deeply that they can't feel pain or anxiety, and keeps them there while the body runs its natural process.

"Is that what your mother wants?"

"Yes. Is this conversation finished?"

We hung up.

I visited her the next day and, while we were alone, asked her if she was ready to die.

"Yes" she whispered.

"If this could be over now, is that what you want?"

"Yes" again.

"Are you ready to go to sleep and not wake up?"

"Please."

The house was still freezing. I could hear workers coming in and out of the front door, trying to get the heater to work. Her nurse and social worker, her paid caregiver, and then someone who identified himself as "her spiritual adviser" arrived. I was the only one in the room who didn't know him. He was young and energetic and had a loud voice, and he had a lot to say. I listened. He talked about God and Jesus and the afterlife. I was glad for the time I'd had alone with her. I leaned down and pressed my cheek to hers when I was leaving.

"I love you," she whispered.

"I love you too."

I went back the next day after the palliative sedation had been started and sat by the patient's side and talked to her. She was deeply asleep, snoring softly, and still she raised one hand into the air and waved.

She died that night. Maybe we'll see her in the waves on the ocean and the clouds in the sky, the way that spiritual adviser fellow said we would. I don't know. I still think of her whenever I drive by the apartment where she lived and died. We're still connected.

Another patient who taught me about connection was an old lady who had a degenerative muscle disease. I was too new to the work to understand the diagnosis that had brought her to hospice, but I could see how helpless she was. Yes, she was bedridden and weak – but she was isolated because she was deaf.

She was in the kind of big nursing home that catches people who need care and don't have any money, the kind of place where there are often bad smells and there always seems to be someone down the hall yelling for help. Her bed was by a window and she watched the squirrels run in the trees and the only time I ever saw her cry was when she told me she'd been left in a dirty diaper for a whole day and no one had come when she pressed her call button for help. She could only hear if I stood inches from her ear and shouted one word at a time. I wondered how it would be to be her, helpless in bed as people appeared and disappeared, mouths moving but no sounds coming out, which was what I saw her caregivers and even my coworkers do.

I learned that when she'd been stronger, she'd zipped around town in her electric wheelchair finding people to talk to and sweet things to eat. Now she was so weak that it was difficult for her to hold a fork or a book and her wheelchair was parked by her bed with a dead battery, taking up space.

She cried out "Ren!" with joy when I entered her room, so of course I visited her often. During my visits I'd putter around, tidying up her area. One day I found a pair of glasses with one lens missing in her bedside drawer. I held them up and asked if she needed them. Yes she did, she answered in the loud voice common to people who can't hear themselves, but they'd been broken for a long time. She was surprised to see them and said how nice it would be to have them again.

Fired up by the idea that an aide had stuck them in that drawer without trying to get them fixed for her, I marched down the hall and demanded that the facility's social worker do something about it. She fired back at me, reminded me that she was responsible for many people and their needs, and said that getting glasses for someone who's bedridden and doesn't have any money can take up to a year. It occurred to me to call the patient's one living friend, a woman so elderly that she could rarely visit; she went to the optometrist the two women had shared and had the broken lens replaced. Then my patient could see again and her world opened up, and I learned something about the kind of advocacy a chaplain can provide. I also learned that if you yell at social workers, they yell right back.

She told me about a book that was on her mind and I found a paperback copy. I'd often arrive for a visit and find her dozing with it lying on the bed in front of her. When she couldn't see regular print any more, I got large print books from the library. Then, as her disease progresssed, she could no longer hold a book and her reading life was over. It had lasted three or four months.

She wanted me to talk about myself, wanted me to teach her about Zen, but yelling one word at a time made that difficult, so instead I sat by her side and asked her to "Tell me a story" and we'd go back to her childhood together. She told me about being a little girl on a farm in the Midwest – I think it was Kansas or Nebraska - with no electricity, no stores or neighbors nearby, and three older brothers to keep up with. She loved her parents. She told me about horse-drawn carts and a cousin with ringlets who gave her hand-me-down dresses, and how amazing ice cream was.

The aides controlled her television. I hated coming into her room and seeing her propped up in front of talk shows she couldn't follow even though they left the sound cranked up to a roar. Finally she and I clicked through the channels until we happened upon the PBS cartoons and over the months she became intimate with *Sesame Street*, *Caillou*, *The Cat in the Hat*, and *Curious George*. She really liked *Curious George*. I put a note on her TV remote saying to leave it on that station. Many afternoons we sat and watched cartoons together.

She wore a ring that had been her mother's. It was gold in an intricate design and had a tiny diamond. One day it was gone. She was extremely upset, calling out over and over, "My ring! My ring!" and waving her bare hand in the air. It was horrible to hear. The ring might have been stolen – yes, that really does happen in nursing homes - or maybe it slipped off of her finger. She continued to mention it for about a month and then it was just another thing that was lost in her past.

And then suddenly, after many months of a gradual decline, she was dying. She became unresponsive and her breathing was labored. She was already wearing oxygen, and I suppose we gave her drugs to help her stay calm. Usually when my people start to die I talk to them, tell them they're safe, tell them they're loved. Because she was deaf, that didn't work, so I sat by her bed, touching her arm, reading and meditating, for most of a day. I'm sure she knew I was there.

People who worked in the facility talked to me about her for years after she died: our friendship was famous in that place.

Where Will I Live

It seems to be a universal hope to remain in our own homes until the day we die. However, as I've mentioned throughout these stories, that often becomes impossible. Whether the diagnosis is cancer, heart failure, or dementia, we'll need help, and we'll only be able to stay in our own home if there's a family member to care for us, or we (or our children) can pay for hired caregivers. If not, we'll have to move to some sort of care facility. I've seen people in luxurious places with staff in clean uniforms and an added (expensive) layer of private paid caregivers by their side while they sleep. I've seen others in really difficult places. And fortunately, for the rest of us, there's a lot of room between those two extremes.

If someone needs help getting up and dressed, someone to do their laundry and cook their meals and maybe feed them, the least expensive solution is what's called a board and care. These look like regular houses from the street, although there may be a wheelchair ramp and an oxygen sign on the door. The maximum number of residents is six and the care is minimal. Residents usually spend the day in front of a television set in the living room, and the caregivers choose the programs which may not be in English; variety shows from the Philippines seem to be quite popular. Caregivers can dispense routine medications but won't be medically trained or licensed, and they may be caring and involved or they may be tired and bored. I've seen gentle ladies in uniforms soothing an upset resident, and I've seen a guy sitting in the kitchen trimming his toenails while an old lady wailed in the dining area. The cost is up and down from $5,000 a month, and Medicare doesn't pay for them, though Medicaid can help.

The large senior living facilities for people who have some money can be very nice. Most residents start in a small private apartment in what's called independent living. Meals are in a dining room and housekeepers come once a week. There are handymen to help with little chores and group activities such as chair exercise and bingo. Days still can be long and I hear my patients complain there's no one to talk to – and yes, some of those dining rooms do look pretty somnolent. When the need increases, the resident will be moved to what's called assisted living and the costs can really rise. Here there's a higher ratio of staff to residents and there's usually someone around who's licensed to dispense serious medications. Activities may be bouncing a balloon in a circle for exercise, watching a movie, or listening to someone read from the paper. Finally, if dementia is developing, the resident may be moved to a memory unit where they will live with other confused people and be watched over by a sizable number of staff – and, again, the cost goes up.

If someone is very sick, they need a skilled nursing facility. Skilled Nursing Facilities will have residents long term, and also people who've just come from a hospital and stay a short time for rehab. This is the only place in which Medicare will pay for room and board, and then there are many complicated hoops to go through for that to happen. Skilled nursing facilities should be the safest, but they're not, and getting into one where there are some sort of activities scheduled, where the food is tasty, and where someone calls when you press your button for help seems to be a matter of luck.

And then there are the county facilities, the beds for people who need long term care and have no money, places like the one I trained in all those years ago. This is the safety net we hear of, and it's both necessary and worn thin. I'm interested in the people who work in these places, the angels who keep showing up even though the building itself is worn down and the staff-to-patient ratio is high. A good nurse can always find a job, and the ones who choose to help the poorest among us have my respect.

For our patients, whether they're in a mansion or a shared room in a facility, that's their home, and that's where we go to care for them.

The county facility in the area where I work was assigned to another chaplain, so I'd never visited there until the social worker asked me to stop by one night when I was on call. She said one of our patients was dying, and his wife – who lived in the same room with him - needed comforting. I went in the early evening. The building felt grim. The walls were a shiny industrial gray and they were scarred where they had been bumped by countless wheelchairs over the years. There was a uniformed guard by the door who showed me where to sign in, inspected my identification, and then gave me the code for the elevator. I wasn't used to elevators that required codes and thought it felt like a prison. It happened that the patient I was visiting was at the end of two long hallways and I saw all of the signs of a care facility that's had its budget cut to the bone but keeps holding on. I passed the nurse's station, but no one was there.

When I found the room I was looking for and walked in, the patient's wife cried out from the bed by the door:

"Can you see if he's still breathing? Can you see if he's dead?"

I turned on a light, went to the side of his bed, and saw a very old man who was doing what we call actively dying, but he was still here. I gave him a blessing, then sat and talked with her, listened to her stories about their marriage and her fears for her future. Periodically as she talked, I walked the few steps across the room and stood by him, hoping that, although he was no longer conscious, he knew he wasn't alone. She was grateful for my company. My duty done, I went home. Several hours later my phone rang: he had died. I drove back to the facility.

When I arrived for the second time that night, as I walked down the long hallway and glanced into the patients' rooms, I saw the way they'd been decorated with posters and strings of lights and heard the murmur of their televisions, and that frightening place felt warmer, more like a long term hotel than a prison. It was a place that offered shelter from the storm for those who most needed it. A nurse was there and she smiled to see me and told me she'd pronounced the time of death and called the mortuary, so I took care of my paperwork, and then went in to see the wife.

Her dead husband's body was still in the bed across the room, now with a sheet pulled over its face, waiting for the undertaker to wheel it away. She was alone and she was crying. I hugged her and pulled a chair next to her and she talked about their marriage — how long it had lasted, what a good husband he had been — and said she didn't know how she could live without him. For the first time, she mentioned a daughter, and I was glad to hear she wasn't alone in the world. I stayed until she was calm, and then I returned home to the safety of my own warm bed.

The next day I went back to see how she was doing. As I parked my car, I saw two women walking from a big Mercedes into the facility. The driver was well dressed and when we rode the elevator together I noticed the diamond that hung from a heavy gold chain around her neck and then, from the two women's conversation, realized this affluent-looking woman was the couple's daughter. I introduced myself and we walked through the hallway to her parents' room. Her mother was alone, and she was still sobbing. I talked about living after a loss and the women listened. I cannot tell you how much difficulty I felt with the difference between the daughter's elegant appearance and the shabbiness of the room her parents had been living in.

The daughter and her friend left the room to find a cup of tea, and her mother turned to me and pleaded with me to talk to her, to say what she was afraid to say herself. "She has an empty bedroom. I could live there. Tell her I'll give her my social security check! Tell her I won't interfere!" I was sure the daughter already knew what her mother wanted, and I had to trust her reasons for leaving the old lady in a place like this.

A few days later, I phoned the daughter and she and I agreed to visit her mother together. The little old lady was in her room, still in her nightgown, quivering with anxiety. Her daughter sat on the empty bed that had been her father's, and leaned back and talked. She told me she had only recently become a widow herself, that her husband had died after a long and harrowing hospitalization. It was a second marriage for both of them, and they had traveled and enjoyed their child-free life together until the day of his heart attack. Their health insurance didn't cover most of his treatments and she'd had to pay out of pocket while she tried to save his life. She described him as a wonderful partner and talked about how she still missed him. So I had thought I would be visiting a widow and a heartless child, and instead found myself with two widows. It crossed my mind that the Mercedes and the diamond might be the last remnants of the daughter's life with her late husband, and they might not reflect the state of her bank account.

I went back to see the patient's wife one more time. I found her in the activity room, wearing a designer dress, sheer black stockings, and beautiful shoes. The other people in the room were wearing sweatpants and t-shirts. She told me her new roommate had taken over her television and was keeping her awake all night watching it with the volume cranked up. She pleaded with me to talk to the roommate just as she had pleaded with me to intervene with her daughter. With the roommate I was able to help; she apologized and promised to keep the volume down.

Years later, I was assigned a patient whose son insisted on keeping his mother in an apartment, even though he was always stressed because he had to work two jobs to pay her rent and her live-in caregivers, and even though the old lady didn't seem to care where she was.

The building he'd put her in was spooky. Some time in the past, it had been a hotel, but a developer had converted it to apartments for seniors. There were large empty public rooms on the ground floor - a library with a pool table, a café, and a bar and restaurant - but I only saw people once or twice and they were at the mailboxes. There were no signs to guide the visitor through the maze of inter-connected buildings and no one to ask for help. I learned to guide myself to the patient's room by using the oversized posters of dead movie stars that decorated the halls: turn right at James Dean and left at Elvis Presley and if you see The Rat Pack, you've gone too far.

On my first visit, when I finally found the door, the woman who answered was young and beautiful, and she was furious. She told me she'd been taking care of the old lady – she gestured at a closed door - for six months, working five days on and two days off. Two weeks ago, the relief person hadn't shown up, and she'd been stuck here without a break. The room we were in had an old dusty deep shag carpet, a television murmuring in the corner, a La-Z-Boy chair so new there were still tags hanging from it, a double mattress on the floor, and a small wooden breakfast table with two chairs. I looked at the jumble of boxes and bags on the kitchen counter and asked how she and the patient were getting food, and she said the old lady's son visited every day. I asked if she couldn't call the agency and have them send a replacement, and learned there was no agency. She was one of the direct caregivers who will take care of someone's parent or child for cash. They may or may not have training and a green card, but bypassing an agency means they make more and the family member pays less.

I asked about the patient. "Oh she's no trouble," she said, "All she does is sleep." Still, she told me, she was fed up. She was leaving at the end of the week, whether the son found a replacement or not.

When I went into the bedroom, I saw the same shag carpet, a chest of drawers, a rolling bedside table, and an old lady in a hospital bed, awake and looking out of the window. I introduced myself and she smiled sweetly. I pulled one of the wooden chairs into the room and sat. The caregiver went back to the mattress on the floor and her cell phone. The patient told me about her life, about her two sons, and about the office she'd worked in when she was young. She seemed glad for the company, and I felt sorry that her caregiver left her so alone, but the old lady didn't complain.

My teammates and I thought she might do well in a board and care home - it would be cheaper for her son than this setup, and might have someone for her to talk to during her long days. But when I met him and suggested this, he blew a gasket. She had lived with his brother for years and then the brother had handed her over to him, and he was going to do it the way he wanted to. He was going to do it even better than his brother had; he was not going to put her in a home. His anger frightened me; I apologized and backed off.

When I visited over the next months, the old lady was always alone in her room, and she always repeated the same story about working in a big building downtown. When I asked about her husband, she said "He was okay" and shrugged. She said her son visited every day and was always angry and worried about money. I talked about how hard he worked to take care of her, and told her this was proof that he loved her, that she was a good mother.

One day I rounded the corner into the hallway that led to the patient's apartment and saw her son and our nurse standing in the doorway. The nurse called out to me; it was so obviously an emergency I thought the patient had died. But no, her son was there because the caregiver hadn't shown up, so he had to leave work and find someone to stay with her. He was as angry as I've ever seen anyone who wasn't actively smashing furniture. The nurse and I checked in with each other and I learned that she, like me, had been coming to do a routine visit and had walked into this. The patient was in her bed, smiling as usual, but she was worried because her son was so angry. I sat with her while we all waited and then, when a woman in a suit and another in a hoodie and low slung jeans arrived to stay with the patient, we left to get on with our days.

For a few months there was a young Chinese woman who was often entertaining her friends when I arrived, and then there was an older woman with a cell phone in her hand and ear buds in place who opened the door and walked back to the mattress on the floor without saying a word.

Once I asked the patient what she did all day while she lay alone in her bed in a silent room. She pointed to an old picture of her parents and their three children and said she spent the day with them. She repeated the story about working downtown every time I visited.

Our social worker eventually found a subsidized bed for her in a skilled nursing home. Her son was glum but worn out from financing the apartment and private care-givers as well as his own home, and he agreed to the move. The patient shrugged. She was cared for, bathed and fed, assessed and visited, for months until she finally, without complaining, died.

I thought about that setup every time I drove by the building she'd been living in. Why, I wondered, did he create such stress for himself by putting her in that strange apartment with a rotating cast of caregivers who mostly seemed to ignore her. It finally occurred to me that his goal might have been to be able to say – to himself and others - that his mother was "at home with private caregivers." Some siblings fight hard to be the "best" child when their parents' life is coming to a close, and maybe he was proving to his mother and his brother that he had won that competition. If so, it must have been hard for him to lose that battle in his own mind, and yet to me he was the good son: he still went to the nursing home to visit her every day.

That woman was unusual because she didn't seem to care where she was. A year or so before I met her, I had a patient who loved her dog and knew she wouldn't be able to take it with her to a nursing home, so she said she'd never move to a facility no matter what happened. She was 84, she lived alone, and she had no friends or family.

When I first visited her, she was so full of energy that it felt like she'd be with us for quite a while. Although she'd lost a lot of weight and she needed help taking care of herself, she could still walk across the room without a cane, and she was certainly able to tell me she didn't care what we thought, didn't want us interfering in her life, and she wasn't ready to die.

She was tiny, not even 5 feet tall, and weighed less than 80 pounds. Her unwashed hair was more brown than gray and had been chopped short so it stuck out at odd angles. She wore a clean old t-shirt and baggy sweatpants. She was barefoot. Her face was lined and worn, and she was missing a few teeth, but that didn't stop her from smiling. Her dog was one of those small long haired mutts that barked when I knocked and then trotted around the room making sure I wasn't dangerous before it hopped up to its place on the old white leather sofa.

Her house looked as if there had been a time when she cared what others thought. She had gone to some trouble to decorate it, anyway. There were crystals in the window, pottery and plastic flowers on the surfaces, and many pictures on the wall, all carefully arranged, all now covered with dust. She pointed out the one that showed a street in the far-away country where she'd been born and when I asked her to tell me about it, she laughed and told me she'd found it in a thrift shop. There was an old copy of *Time* magazine on the coffee table with a portrait of Trump on the cover. I commented on it, and she told me how much she liked him. "He's a business man!" she said proudly.

I like to get close, so I pulled a straight chair next to her lounger. She scolded me and said to get it off the carpet. I moved it back and spoke more loudly, listened more carefully as we talked. If she wouldn't let me next to her physically, I'd have to work harder to establish a bond.

On that first visit, even as her body was wasting away, she was still able to talk nonstop, to start to answer the question asked and then to veer off into complicated stories of anger and blame.

I asked about family.

"Oh those people are gone. I was married three times, you know, and my last mother-in-law said she was surprised I kept his name, but I kept visiting her. I liked her. He – the husband – was a bum. She and I agreed. We always talked what a bad husband he'd been. And relatives, I don't know, relatives they were all left behind when I came to this country and I never saw them again. Not any of them. Sometimes I tried to find some of them but I guess it was too late. I guess they didn't care. Well okay then I don't care either, they're history and I've done a good job of taking care of myself here."

She insisted she didn't need family or friends, but I knew she was going to need us. Caregivers from social services came for two hours mornings and nights, and our social worker had told her she couldn't get any more in-home care unless she could pay for it, which she couldn't, so she would need to move to a nursing home. When our social worker had brought this up, she'd refused to even think about it. She said she wouldn't leave her dog.

As her health failed and she needed more care, it would be just her and that dog for long days and nights. She'd lose control of her bladder and bowels. She'd need to get food, and to take the right pill at the right time. Eventually, for her own safety, she'd have to move to a place where her physical symptoms could be monitored and treated, and there was nothing here that said that would go smoothly. She was going to be a problem. At least I succeeded in getting her approval in that visit. She told me to come back any time, and I agreed.

The week after our first meeting, I was looking at my list of patients and I thought about visiting her again. I was taking a new social worker on my visits that day, showing her how we work in hospice so, when space opened up in my afternoon, I sent her a message to meet me at the patient's house. When she parked her car behind mine and walked toward me, I saw a short Chinese woman wearing generic black polyester pants and sensible shoes. She was enthusiastic. She told me she had experience in social work but was new to hospice and home visits. I liked her. I told her about myself, that I'd been doing this work for some years, and that there was more to spiritual care than saying a prayer. We walked to the patient's house together, and I pointed at the eccentric arrangement of mostly dead plants and broken furniture in the front yard. We smiled.

I knocked on the door and then pushed it open when there was no answer. I called the patient's name, and then turned toward the sound of her dog whimpering. My patient was lying on the floor on her side, her arms outstretched, with the dog huddled in the curve of her legs. She wore only a t-shirt, and the sight of her naked hipbone was startling. A little bowl had been knocked over and matchbooks were scattered on the floor by her head. I stepped over an electric cord, wondering if she had tripped on it, and then over her legs. I kneeled by her side. Her eyes were partially open, staring at nothing. I touched her shoulder, surprised by the warmth of her skin, shook her gently, called her name. There was no response. The dog remained silent, watching.

I turned to the new social worker and asked,

"Do you know how to find a pulse?" She shook her head No.

I called the patient's name more loudly and shook her harder, trying to wake her. I put my fingers on her neck. I didn't feel a heartbeat. I turned to the social worker.

"I think she might be dead."

I was too stunned to think clearly. I finally remembered that I could call my company's triage nurse, the one who's always on the other end of the phone to help in emergencies. She told me to put my hand on the patient's chest and see if it was rising and falling. I did. I told her it wasn't moving. That was all she needed to know. She said she'd send someone out to pronounce the time of death and hung up.

The new social worker watched while I took a blanket off the sofa and covered the body. The dog made a nest in it and settled back down. The new social worker and I looked at each other. There we were, together in a small untidy room with a dead body in the corner.

"This doesn't usually happen" I told her.

I kept waiting for the patient to sit up and laugh at me for making such a foolish mistake, but she never did. The triage nurse sent out an email announcing the death, and the patient's nurse called to say she was starting another visit and would be there in about an hour to make the death pronouncement. I was amazed she wasn't dropping everything to rush right over. Then I realized – she didn't have to hurry, because our patient wasn't going anywhere.

Usually when someone dies, we call the family and the mortuary, but there was no one to call for this lady. The new social worker had called her boss and handed the phone to me. I described the scene and the boss said she'd call the coroner to take care of the body.

I gave the phone back to the new social worker and told her, "You know this means we're bonded forever" and she nodded solemnly.

Then I realized the dog was a problem. The lady had mentioned her landlord and I thought he could help, so my coworker stayed with the body while I left to knock on neighbors' doors to try to find his phone number.

I'd recovered from my shock, and it felt great to have something to do. First I tried the little house to the south, but no one answered. Next I tried the larger house to the north, the one with the warning sign and the barking dog behind a chain link fence. A voice called from behind the closed door.

"Who are you!"

"I'm the chaplain visiting your neighbor. I'm sorry to say she has died, and I'm trying to find the landlord's name. Might you have it?"

He shouted at the dog to stop barking and then there was a pause, some sounds from inside, and finally he opened the door a few feet. He was a nice looking young guy, a little frowsy like maybe he'd been enjoying a nap or even an afternoon joint when I interrupted him. He gave me a piece of paper with the landlord's name and number, and also told me the lady in the house across the street with the Honda in the driveway might be able to help.

Now I was feeling good: this detective work was paying off. So when I knocked on the door of the lady across the street, I was energized and smiling. When I told her the patient was dead, she was shocked and sad.

Finally, we'd arrived at sadness. I slowed down. We talked.

The neighbor knew what she'd been seeing. We agreed there might be a silver lining as the patient's quality of life was so diminished and her future had been so precarious. She told me she'd sometimes helped with the dog and, though she couldn't take it permanently, she could take care of it for a few days while things were being sorted out. She came across with me and as we entered the living room, I smiled at the new social worker and she smiled back broadly, relieved at the progress we'd made. The neighbor looked at the patient quietly for a minute and then found a leash and put it on the little dog. The dog wouldn't move. It whimpered, pulled against the leash, and insisted on staying where it was. She unhooked it and the dog curled back against the patient's body.

I dialed the landlord's number and left a message. He called me back within minutes, and told me he would take the dog, that this had been the arrangement all along. He said he'd be there soon. Then the neighbor left and joined the small cluster of people on the sidewalk. One of them called out to me, "Did you call 911?"

I explained the patient hadn't wanted resuscitation, that she'd signed a piece of paper that was posted by the door so there was nothing for 911 to do, and so we were waiting for the coroner. The social worker and I smiled at each other again. We were back in control.

Time passed. The new social worker left. The landlord came, we talked about the lady, and I was relieved when the dog went with him willingly. The neighbors standing on the sidewalk talked themselves out and went home. The sun moved across the living room wall. My energy faded from the adrenaline rush. I was alone with my patient and could talk to her, tell her how glad I was I'd found her, that I felt she'd summoned me, that I was sure the landlord would take good care of the dog, and that by dying this way she'd just avoided a whole lot of end-of-life suffering.

Then the coroner came, and I was done. I'll never know why she fell or what caused her death.

She was the norm in wanting to stay in her own home, and she had the little dog as an excuse for her determination. I had another patient who seemed to be doing well in her apartment with the same arrangement of caregivers from social services coming to help for two hours in the morning and two hours in the evening, but she was the one who said she had to move into a facility.

She was the kind of person people wanted to help. Her tiny body was twisted and she was in pain, but she always smiled. When she was alone during the day, she rolled around her subsidized apartment in her wheelchair, listening to public radio, microwaving soup, and reading Mary

Oliver poems. Her apartment had a view into a birch tree, and she sat in silence watching the birds.

After I'd been visiting her for months, talking about her difficult life, about Buddhism and forgiveness, she said she had grown too weak to be alone and she needed to move to a nursing home. I dreaded what this would mean. I argued with her, saying she'd be better off staying where she was, that nursing homes were noisy and unpleasant. She said she'd be fine: all she needed was to be able to see a tree and maybe go outside once in a while.

Two social workers began making calls, one from our company and another from an outside agency, and they couldn't find a bed anywhere. Each nursing home allocates a number of beds to Medicare/Medi-Cal patients, and getting one is a matter of luck and timing. Finally, though no one told me this directly, it seemed someone taught her how to play the game: since most of the subsidized beds went to people who were being discharged from hospitals, if she wanted one, she would have to go through a hospital to get it. Hospice is for people who are dying, and hospitals are for people who are trying to live. So when she went to the Emergency Room in an ambulance, she was automatically discharged. That meant I could no longer visit her on company time – and yet I went to see her that day. She looked even smaller in the hospital bed, and for the first time she wasn't friendly and welcoming. She was frightened. We both wondered what would become of her.

It was just coincidence that I was sitting by her side when two middle-aged women with clipboards, both in black suits and high heels, entered the room. These were the hospital administrators, making their morning rounds. She couldn't stay in the hospital, they said, but a bed was available in the nursing home down the street, one where I'd visited patients many times. It was suddenly so simple.

But then, when I asked what kind of room she'd be in, they said she'd have the middle bed in a three-bed room. I knew this meant she would be hemmed in by curtains on either side; she'd have only a small chest of drawers to hold her possessions; her only view would be of the wall, and she'd hear the noise from her neighbors' televisions, day and night.

"Might she upgrade to a double room after a while?" I asked.

They saw my badge. They knew who I was. Their smiles said they knew I already knew the answer when they said "No." The beds in the nicer double rooms were kept for people who could pay.

Then one of the women looked up from her clipboard and said, "But there is a bed in one of the big rooms with four beds." In theory, a room with four beds was worse than one with three. But I had seen those rooms and knew they were large and a wall of windows made them bright. I told the ladies in suits we were interested, and they arranged for me to visit the nursing home on the spot.

The available bed was next to a sliding glass door, looking out on an inner courtyard full of trees and plants. "She'll take it!" I promised, and snapped a picture with my phone so my patient could see her new home. When I walked back to the hospital and showed it to her, she cried with relief. One of our social workers made an extra effort to get her readmitted to hospice, and by the end of the day she was in her new subsidized home.

She lived there until she died months later. She became friends with the other patients and their visitors, and sat in the sun listening to her radio over headphones. She organized her area so a book of poetry was at hand, and care-givers and friends made sure she always had a flower to look at. I visited often, and she never forgot to express her joy at living in that place. People all over the country were praying for her. I wondered if maybe that's why she got so lucky.

Making Plans

Many – no, actually most - of us seem to assume that we'll live long and happy lives until a day in the distant future when we'll die peacefully in our sleep. We don't think or talk about what we might want if things go in a different direction, even though the chances are good they will.

If we get sick, whether it's a fast-moving cancer or a glacially slow dementia, we'll probably reach a point where we can't speak for ourselves. When that happens, someone will need to make medical decisions for us. This person becomes known as a DPOA (because they have the Durable Power of Attorney for healthcare) and the form they work from is called an advance directive. Unless we've filled out the form and chosen who we want to speak for us, the closest family member will carry that burden, and, if they don't have any guidance, they always agree to extreme measures.

When I was training in the hospital, I became friends with an elderly couple. He had picked up an infection during a routine knee replacement, and now he lived in a hospital bed receiving antibiotics and she lived sitting at his side keeping him company. One night he had some sort of crisis and was whisked into the ICU. His wife and I stood over his unconscious body the next day and I asked her what his wishes were. She admitted they'd never talked about it: "I only know he wouldn't want to be on life support," she said, not knowing that was exactly what she was seeing. He was eventually stabilized so he could return to a regular hospital bed, and then a meeting was called with several doctors, his surgeon, and the palliative care team. I was allowed to attend too. The medical jargon flowed freely while the doctors talked and the old lady listened. Finally the palliative care doctor explained what comfort care would mean – no more medical interventions, all care aimed at quality of life - and I watched and listened, hoping she would say yes. Just as she seemed to be ready to accept that it would be best to let her husband live the days he had left in peace, the surgeon spoke: "Well, there is one more operation we could try – it's risky, but it might work" and that was that. The wife grasped at this straw, and the patient, already old and weak, went through still another procedure. He never regained consciousness and died days later in an acute care hospital bed. If the two of them had been able to talk about what he wanted when he first went in for the routine surgery that started his downward spiral, weeks of suffering and expense could have been avoided for both of them.

Years later, working in hospice, I visited a couple in their 50s who were living in a house that was beautiful, dark, and silent. The wife sat with me in the living room. She told me that her husband's doctor was a friend of theirs, and, unforgettably, said "If he had just told us the truth – if we'd known how bad the cancer was, we would have done it differently. He kept encouraging us to try something else, so the last year was spent going in and out of the hospital and none of it did any good. We could have been enjoying each other and the life we had left and instead we lost that time and now he's dying."

I remember the woman whose mother was lost in dementia who said "She never would have wanted to live like this." The patient was in a care home, either asleep or crying out for help, and the daughter visited nearly every day. She demanded antibiotics when the old lady got another urinary tract infection, and brought cases of nutritional supplements for the caregivers to give her, all designed to prolong the poor woman's life. Her mother hadn't made an advance directive and the daughter was afraid of what other family members would say if she didn't do everything she could to keep the unfortunate woman alive. If her mother had been able to talk with her before her dementia was advanced, if she could have given her daughter permission to let her go when it reached this point, both of them would have been released from this endless non-life.

I had another patient whose family had the money to keep her in the memory unit of a nice facility. When she came on our service, her dementia was so advanced that she was unable to speak or care for herself in any way. Her husband hired private caregivers to get her up and in a wheelchair in the morning, and take her to the dining room where they'd spend up to three hours coaxing her to take just one more bite of baby food, one more sip of Ensure. This is not that unusual. What was unusual was, the patient had seen her mother go through the same thing and so, when she could still speak for herself, she had asked her husband to stop feeding her when her life reached the point that it had no meaning. After she'd been on our service for a little over a year, he said that time had come. The couple's children agreed and he finally let her attendants leave her in bed to die peacefully. It didn't take long. She had made her plans, and he'd done what she asked, out of love.

It's hard for anyone to say whether another's life has meaning, to judge that elusive element we call "quality of life." One of my patients told her children that no one should try to feed her if she reached the point where she could no longer feed herself. I liked that so much, I put it in my own advance directive.

Then there was a difficult case of a woman who made plans, had them drawn up by a lawyer, asked someone to take on the responsibility of her care if she reached a point when she could no longer speak for herself, and was still kept alive in exactly the way she'd tried to avoid.

I heard about her from my coworkers before I went to see her. They said she was aggressive and causing problems in the nursing home, that she screamed and threw things at staff members when they tried to clean her. There was a feeding tube attached to her stomach surgically and she pulled at it until it came free of the bag hanging by her bed. Its milky liquid puddled on the floor, making more work for the staff. The two other women in the three-bed room, strangers to her, were complaining about the commotion, and the nurses and aides were unhappy too.

As I approached her for the first time, I saw the rails on her bed were up, and they were cushioned so she wouldn't hurt herself. She looked at me, made a terrible noise, and waved her arms wildly. Nurses and aides walked by without turning their heads. I'm supposed to comfort people, not upset them, so I left.

A week later, the whole team was called to a meeting by the facility staff. Her decision-maker was a very large man in a wheelchair with long gray hair and an impressive beard. A thin young woman with dangling earrings sat beside him. As we introduced ourselves, I learned he was the patient's pastor, and the woman with him was his translator. She explained that he, and all of the members of his congregation, including our patient, was deaf. No one — not in my company's notes or in the nursing home — had mentioned this.

The pastor told us the patient had been living alone when she had a stroke a year ago. A neighbor had called 911 and she was taken to the ER, where the doctors had inserted a feeding tube to keep her alive. Now the doctors had said there was an infection around the insertion site, and the tube needed to be removed. The pastor said he understood that taking out the tube meant the patient would die, and he said he was sure this was what she would have wanted. He even said a really good prayer to end our meeting.

I looked into her room on my way out of the nursing home, and saw that a sign had been tacked over her bed saying DEAF, so at least people like me weren't appearing at her bedside and babbling into her silence. There was a picture board on the dresser so she could point to words – "yes," "no," "hot," "cold," "pain," but I never knew whether she was able to use it. At least it felt as if we'd made progress.

A few days later, the nursing home called and told us the pastor was out of the picture. When the patient had been moved there, he'd been with her and so they had been talking to him -- but they'd just learned he wasn't the legal decision maker. The patient had given that responsibility to a cousin years earlier. There's a lot of talk about patient privacy and being careful who we give information to, so it was startling that we'd all been talking to the wrong person. I never heard anything more about it.

The hospice nurse phoned the cousin, and then asked me to help. It was a busy time, so I grabbed a few moments between appointments and dialed her number while I sat in my car in a parking lot one afternoon. She answered, and I closed my eyes so I could concentrate and hear her story. She said that the patient's lawyer had sent her the advance directive years earlier, and when it had arrived in the mail, she'd read it and then filed it away carefully. They had never talked about it, but she knew it said the patient didn't want to be on life support.

When the patient was in the emergency room a year earlier, the doctors had called and asked if they could insert a feeding tube through her nose "just for a few days, to see if it would help." She was persuaded, and she agreed. The patient tried to pull the tube out. The doctors had then asked the cousin to allow them to surgically insert a feeding tube into her stomach "just to see if it would help" and it had kept her alive, bedridden, and entirely dependent on strangers for her most basic needs, for nearly a year. Now the patient was failing, and a different set of doctors had told the cousin they wanted to take the feeding tube out.

I want to say that again, to underscore what just happened in this story. Although the patient had left written instructions saying she didn't want to be on life support, the relative she had chosen to speak for her had been persuaded to ignore the patient's wishes by doctors who she never even met. And now a different group of doctors were telling the cousin to remove the feeding tube, acknowledging this would cause her death.

The cousin told me she'd talked to her priest and he'd said the church does not condemn withdrawing artificial life support. Her priest had even connected her with someone higher up in the diocese who'd studied the matter more deeply, and he too gave her permission to accept the doctors' advice.

By then, I knew we'd been talking for quite a long time and was worried I'd be late for my next appointment. I thought the authority of the church could settle the matter and I could finish our conversation, so I said,

"It must be such a relief to have their approval."

The cousin agreed but said she was still not comfortable with it. It was still nagging her. She couldn't say yes.

I forced myself to put aside my worry about time and concentrate on her again. She spoke at length of the difficulty of knowing she was doing the right thing.

"It's such a responsibility," I tried, and she agreed. In fact, she reminded me, the patient's wishes were clearly spelled out and she was fulfilling them, and still she was uneasy, worried, upset. I said I'd heard about this difficulty from other people. I told her I'd heard that instead of feeling they were helping someone have a natural death, they felt as if they were murdering them.

She jumped on the word. She said that was exactly it, and I was the first person who'd dared to come out and say it. I think that was when she began to trust me, a stranger who was sitting in a parking lot and talking to her over a car speaker.

We talked about the way in which the patient appeared to be suffering, how she'd been stuck in a hospital bed for nearly a year now.

I said "Not eating or drinking is a way that people have been dying for centuries. The doctors say dying people don't feel hunger the way we do, and that this is a comfortable end of life."

"It's just so hard" she answered, and then I realized what was missing.

"This is love in action," I told her. "Real love isn't always comfortable and easy. Real love can be very hard work." That's when she began crying. That's what she'd been looking for. She repeated this several times.

"Love is hard work."

I suggested she write the words down so she wouldn't forget them. She said she wouldn't need to. She hadn't thought of what might happen when she agreed to be her cousin's medical decision maker, and she had been afraid to follow those written wishes when her cousin needed her. Now she would be able to.

The tube was removed that week, and the patient was finally allowed the death she had asked for when she filled out her advance directive so many years earlier. I called the cousin after the death and she was doing fine. In my view, that patient had really bad luck, and she's one of the reasons I jump on the chance to tell people to not just fill out an advance directive but to have a conversation to with the person they've asked to speak for them, to make sure that person understands what they want and is willing to see that they get it.

I had another patient who made no plans at all, and who got very lucky at the end. She had no family, but she was still at home because she had friends who were caring for her. When I called to set up a visit, it was one of those friends who answered. She told me that she and her sister lived across the country and were visiting when they found the patient in distress. They'd been caring for her ever since. She warned me they weren't religious, but said they needed help and they'd like to see me.

When I knocked on the door the next day, a middle aged woman opened it. Her clothes were rumpled, and she looked tired and worried. I could see an old lady lying in a hospital bed behind her. She lay quietly, her white hair a puff of cotton on her pillow, her body barely a bump under the blankets. She opened her eyes and smiled. As I was telling her I was the chaplain from hospice, a second woman appeared in the kitchen doorway and beckoned to me with such urgency that I thought I'd done something wrong. Some people ask us not to use the word *hospice* around the patient, and I wondered whether this was one of them.

Everything in the kitchen was neat and tidy except for a piece of plywood covering a broken window pane. One of the women closed the door and they told me their story. The patient had been their teacher. They had moved away years ago, but had stopped by to see the old lady and bring her a gift of a bag of groceries when they were in town for a high school reunion. There was no answer when they knocked at the front door, so they had come around to the side of the house, peered in the window, and discovered her lying on the kitchen floor. She hadn't opened her eyes when they knocked, so they'd called 911. The firemen who responded had broken the window to get inside, put the unconscious woman on a stretcher, and taken her to the emergency room. The sisters followed in their rental car, their gift of groceries forgotten on the kitchen counter.

At the hospital, doctors gave the patient fluids and ran tests, and when she woke, she and her friends learned that she had an untreated breast cancer that had spread through her body. The doctors said a cure was impossible, and that going home on hospice would be her best option. The old lady had agreed; the doctors had turned to the sisters at her side and asked them to sign some forms, and suddenly they found themselves responsible for a dying woman. The hospital social worker told them there was no trace of the old lady in the system. She had no health insurance, not even Medicare.

A week had passed. My company had sent a nurse who gave them a number to call if they needed help. The old lady didn't need much; she didn't complain, and slept most of the time. They gave her some medicine according to the nurse's directions; some sips of water, thickened so she wouldn't choke; and a diaper change twice a day. The patient could only smile and nod, and whisper yes or no to their questions. The landlady lived next door, and she had stopped by and thanked them. This was all much more than they'd bargained for when they visited with a gift for their old teacher.

They told me that the hospice social worker – my coworker - had gone through piles of papers looking for tax returns or bank statements so she could begin the process of either finding the patient a bed in a nursing home or hiring caregivers to stay with her, but all she found was a shoe box containing $2,000 in cash. She had told the sisters she'd try to find her a safe place where she'd be cared for, but without money or health insurance, it would take a very long time.

They didn't have a long time. They needed to go home. That was why the woman had beckoned me with such urgency: they wanted me to help them tell the patient they were leaving the next day.

We agreed I would start the conversation with the patient, and then they would talk to her. As we approached, the patient opened her eyes and smiled. I reminded her I was the chaplain, that I was here to help, and said her friends needed to speak with her. She nodded. I stood aside while they told her they loved her but they had to go home. They told her that, since she couldn't care for herself, the hospice company would find her a bed in a nursing home. I thought to myself that this was unlikely, but kept quiet. The patient nodded; she never stopped smiling. She whispered her thanks to them. I said a short prayer for the old lady's benefit, and the sisters and I hugged and parted. They were crying with relief.

When I called my company's social worker later and asked about the case, she was angry. She said it had taken her hours to go through all of the papers in the patient's desk, only to learn she had nothing. She said those hours had been wasted and she called the patient irresponsible. She said finding a bed was time consuming enough when a patient was already on Medicare; it would be nearly impossible for this lady, and she didn't have the time to sit on hold with government agencies. I said I guessed the old lady had lived her life on a cash basis and that's why she'd never filed for Social Security or Medicare. The social worker said she was too busy to think about it.

Our hospice company couldn't leave the patient helpless and alone, so we sent nurses' aides to stay in the house after the sisters left. Usually Medicare would reimburse the company for these employees' time, but this woman would be a rare charity case. I visited her once more, but there wasn't much for me to do. It had been the sisters who had needed me, not the patient.

The lucky old lady was comfortable; she died in her own home within a week. She had done nothing to plan for her future, hadn't even seen a doctor, and she'd been saved from dying alone on the kitchen floor, or in a nursing home among strangers, by chance visitors.

Her landlady called a couple of months later and asked me to stop by. When I did, she gave me a check made out to the hospice company. She had sold the patient's belongings, and she wanted to donate the money to us. She showed me the figures she'd written on the back of an envelope, money in and money out, and I said it looked good and thanked her. She told me how fond she'd been of the patient, how she'd kept her in the house at under-market rent for decades as a kind of good luck charm. We cried together, maybe from sorrow but also from relief that she had died so well.

That lady seemed to have good luck. But then I had a patient who had worked and invested her money, planned carefully and met with lawyers and got everything set up so she could stay in the home she was so proud of with the cat she loved, and then died drugged and alone in a facility, cared for by strangers. She was stubborn and she had bad luck.

I liked her the first time she opened her door and smiled at me. She was birdlike, small and thin, and her hair, which appeared to be dyed, puffed around her head like a crown of feathers. She was wearing pink cotton pants and a lavender t-shirt, and, although there were food stains on her clothes, she'd taken the trouble to tie a silk scarf around her neck. She held herself stiffly and moved slowly as she led me into the small living room. She seemed vulnerable.

The house was simple, a two bedroom bungalow with a big backyard in what had become a fancy neighborhood. Her furniture looked as if it was left over from someone's college days except for the pretty French Provincial chair she sat in – but even that had a sunken seat and had been shredded by the cat. There were books everywhere. I sat on one of those foam slab couches, but within minutes I began to wheeze from cat hair and dust, so I pulled a straight chair from the breakfast nook for myself.

There was one surprise: she had a beautiful baby grand piano. Of course it was the first thing I asked about. She smiled and said she'd bought it because she wanted to play Mozart. Then she asked me what it meant to be a chaplain.

"Hospice is comfort care, and chaplains are included in the team to be sure you're comfortable spiritually as well as physically. My work is spiritual, not religious. I'm ordained as a Zen Buddhist priest, and I do this work as a way of bringing my vow into the world."

I was ready to say more, but she was satisfied and ready to talk about herself. She was more interested in her story than mine. She had left her parents' home, put herself through college, learned a skill, got a job, saved her money, and bought this little house. She'd never stopped her quarrel with her mother who was now dead many years. She had never married and she was used to taking care of herself. She had developed a drinking problem and got sober in AA, and still prayed to the God she'd found there. An old co-worker was helping her keep track of her bills, and she trusted him to make medical decisions for her too.

She'd had breast cancer several years before, had endured many rounds of chemotherapy and radiation, and it had gone into remission. That's when she had bought the piano. Now a new cancer had formed and her oncologist told her she should go on hospice. That's what was confusing to her: she insisted the cancer was gone, and she thought whatever pain she felt from the lump in her chest must be coming from something else. The oncologist had given her drugs but she refused to take them. She said she knew herself better than the doctors did and asked whether I knew a good osteopath.

"You're on hospice because you have cancer," I'd say. "The doctor has tried all of the possible treatments but there's nothing more he can do. To qualify you for hospice services, he's said you probably have six months or less to live, although of course no one knows for sure. Hospice is a service that makes it possible for you to stay in your home. It's free, a Medicare benefit. All of these visitors, any equipment you need, and all of the drugs are free. You're an example of what it's designed for, to let people stay in their own homes when they're nearing the end of life."

She'd nod and blink. I could practically see the wheels turning in her mind as she tried to make sense of this. Then she'd change the subject. She could only see the life she'd created, not the one that was happening to her, and in the life she had created, she had cured cancer. In her stubbornness, that was the end of the story.

I visited once a week. I enjoyed her and thought I could help her understand what was happening. I didn't want death to be a surprise when it came for her.

I praised her for having taken such good care of herself. She blinked her eyes like a little bird, then pointed out the French door to the garden she'd had installed in her bedroom, and reminded me she'd also remodeled the kitchen. She would smile. She was proud of herself for taking out a second mortgage on the house, in case she needed money now that she was older.

I asked whether she was still playing the piano. I noticed the sheet music didn't change, and dust was accumulating on the keyboard cover, but she always said she was. I asked whether she was still driving the old Corolla that was parked in the driveway, but she always said she wasn't. She did admit that she'd begun taking the pain pills prescribed by the doctor she didn't like.

Then she began falling. One morning our home health aide found her lying on the bathroom floor, bruised and shivering from the cold. When I came to see her she said "Anyone can fall" and laughed it off. I asked her to remember to wear her Medic Alert when she got up in the night and she said she always did, but it had been lying useless on the bedside table when she fell.

A month or so later, she was wearing it when she fell again, and the medics who answered the call took her to the emergency room. Again she was badly bruised but no bones were broken. The hospital social worker said she couldn't go home alone, so there was a woman from an agency in the house the next time I visited. She seemed hesitant, almost apologetic. I introduced myself, showed her my badge, and went into the bedroom where the patient was sitting in a nest of blankets, with books and food scattered around her. She shrugged off her fall, showed me what she was reading and said she liked staying in bed. The caregiver appeared in the doorway and looked at us. The patient told her to go away and leave her alone. She made a face at her when she left.

Days after that visit, she called me. She had found the notes the paid caregivers kept — when and how much she ate, her sleeping patterns, her trips to the bathroom — and she was outraged, mortified, and demanding to know why they were spying on her. I tried to explain. "Those are the caregivers that are there to keep you safe. You need them. They're just doing their job. Have you eaten? Please be nice to them. I'm afraid you'll fall again."

The next time I visited, she had fired the caregivers; she was alone. The house was messy and she looked disheveled. She admitted she'd forgotten to feed the cat and then that she'd forgotten to feed herself. I hovered behind her as she walked to the kitchen, leaning on the door jamb, then a chair, then the piano, then the wall. She pulled a little berry pie out of the refrigerator and I held it for her as she furniture-walked back to bed. While we talked, she took two bites and then set it aside. She said a neighbor was coming to take care of the cat's overflowing litter box. She insisted she was doing fine.

When I left the house, I called the doctor and told her the patient had fired the caregivers and was alone, and I didn't think she was safe. She pointed out that the patient was walking and talking and feeding herself, and said she could still make her own decisions. I wasn't so sure about that. I saw her confusion and fragility. She called her "a strong, independent woman." She said we should just visit often to keep an eye on her.

A week later, when I rang the bell at the usual time, I could hear movement inside. I rang the bell again, and then turned the knob and called her name.

She was in the back bedroom, teetering as she bent to retrieve her cane from under the desk. She was wearing a pink flowered nightgown and her hair was matted and uncombed. She'd stopped dyeing it, and her roots were showing. She turned to look up at me and smiled as if she'd been caught and didn't want to be scolded.

"Look," she said brightly, pulling the cane to her side, "I've tied a red scarf to it so I can find it when I need it."

We moved to the living room. She was alert that day, and eager to talk about her fury with a neighbor who had sneaked over one night and disconnected her car battery after she side-swiped a parked truck. The neighbor said she was worried about neighborhood kids walking to and from school, but she insisted there were no kids in the area when she'd had her accident and anyway said the accident was the truck driver's fault for parking the way he did. She talked about the bills that had been accumulating and needed her attention. The one from the caregiving agency bothered her a lot. She was caught in a loop on the subject and went on and on about it, filling the air with her anxiety.

I listened and then finally I interrupted her. "You know, I'm the chaplain. When your friend comes later, he can help sort out your bills. I understand these are nagging problems, but I wonder if there's anything else you'd like to talk about with me while I'm here. My allergy to your cat seems to come and go, and today I can already feel it. So let's talk while we can. Tell me what else is going on. When I phoned you earlier in the week, you said your health was getting worse."

"Yes, this tumor in my chest is growing. It really hurts when it gets bumped so I always have to be careful." She went through her medical history again. But this time, as she repeated the story of the first and then the second cancer, there was something new at the end of the story. She said:

"And then I'm going to die."

I was amazed. For six months I had worried she couldn't understand that death was drawing near. Today, for the first time, she had shown me that she did.

I agreed with her. "That's probably the case. And we want to make sure you're comfortable and safe until that happens."

I urged her to not waste these precious days in anger and anxiety. I reminded her she could trust her God. We talked about finding gratitude for the life we have rather than getting lost in yearning for the life we've lost. We talked about not getting stuck in negative thinking, about not getting on the train of thoughts when they turn dark, and about setting aside worries about things like paying bills. She listened, nodded, and agreed. She thanked me. She agreed to take life one day at a time.

I'd been there for over an hour. My breathing had become raspy and my chest felt tight. I said I was sorry, but I had to leave. She stayed on the rigid foam sofa as we said our goodbyes, her feet pulled up and her nightgown pulled over her knees like a little kid.

It was a relief to get out of the house, to breathe the cold clean winter air, to let go of the strain of trying to find the right thing to say.

Two hours later she phoned my office, panicked and screaming. The nurse who answered the phone tried to tell her which drug she should take, but she couldn't sort through her shoe box of pill bottles to find it. She didn't stop screaming. One of our nurses went to her house and gave her something, and stayed with her while she slept.

It scared us, and it scared her so much that the next day she agreed to let us help her move to a facility. I visited her there that afternoon and she was sitting up in bed in the same pink nightgown, smiling, accepting the help that was offered, and delighted by the attention she was getting. I was so relieved to see her safe.

But the panic returned later that night and she began screaming again. For her sake, and the sake of the sleep of the other patients, the doctor gave her stronger drugs. She quieted and slept. She never woke again.

She died some days later. She had created a life, lived it, and then lost control of it. It would have been different if she'd died in her own home, understanding and accepting what was happening. That was what I wanted for her. But she refused to admit that she needed help, couldn't bear having strangers in her house and was outraged by their cost, so she died in a drugged sleep in a facility. It was stubbornness, and it was bad luck.

Or maybe when she told me she knew death was coming, I should have stayed and talked about it more. Maybe I missed something. The nurse on staff said the patient had tried to call me before she'd called the hospice number. Our doctor said probably something had happened — maybe she had a stroke — that caused her death. I'll never know whether she was screaming from physical or emotional pain, and I wondered what else I could have done to help this woman who I'd liked so much.

She had bad luck in spite of her plans, but there are also people who seem to make their own bad luck. In one spectacular example of this, an old man lived alone and had come to our service after he called 911 for help one night. The paramedics had found him lying on his bed, unable to get up to feed, bathe or toilet himself. That started the wheels of social services grinding, and those wheels ended at hospice.

The front door was unlocked, and after I knocked, I pushed it open. I entered a small room with wall to wall bookshelves. And the books were good: literature, history, art. I was hopeful. I'm always looking for patients who I can have a conversation with. I entered his bedroom smiling, looking forward to meeting this intellectual with a vaguely familiar name. I introduced myself as usual, "Hello, my name is Ren and I'm the chaplain."

"Get out!" he hollered.

I kept trying. "I'm not here to push God or religion. I'm here because hospice is about comfort, and that includes both the physical and the non-physical."

"Get out!" he hollered again.

I left. I was taught in training that sometimes the chaplain is the only person the patient can throw out of the room. They can be rude to a doctor or a nurse, but they have to let them in. Not the chaplain. I was taught that throwing me out may be the only control the patient has left over their life.

I found the binder where I record my visit on a shelf below more books, and saw the books were about Zen. There was a good three feet of them. I signed my name and then, just in case, stuck my head through the door into his room.

"Could I just say one more thing?"

"GET OUT."

An online search showed he was a mildly famous 60's radical and author, and I felt like he missed something that day. If he was so alone that he had to call 911 when he needed help, I might have at least been a little company.

I meet a lot of lonely people. It's not that unusual. Their days are filled by going to a job, coming home and eating alone, watching television until bedtime, not complaining, not grasping for more. I remember one man like this who had gone to the doctor with a persistent cough and been sent home with a diagnosis of terminal cancer. He was in his 70's.

His apartment was small and the carpet and paint were worn. After he opened the door for me for the first time, he sat in a worn Ikea chair that faced a television sitting on a box. I pulled a wooden chair from the kitchenette to visit with him.

I asked about family. He'd never married and his parents and brother were dead. He told me he did have a nephew who'd said he would help when the time came. It was an awkward conversation. I thought he wasn't used to talking to ladies. I kept trying to do my assessment, wanting to find out what I could do to help. He answered in one and two syllables.

Then there was a knock on the door: it was the nephew, arriving much sooner than the patient had expected him. After an enthusiastic greeting, the young man went into the other room to clean up from the trip. The patient turned to me and said "I never expected this" and his face was full of joy.

I visited the two of them a few more times before he died; neither of them had much to say to me. I wasn't a part of this story, just an observer of a happy outcome. The nephew brought connection with him and the patient received it gratefully. He was another one who had made no plans but he had good luck.

When I was in my first few months of training in the hospital, I had a wonderful patient who I visited every day, a little old lady from the Philippines who was a devout Catholic. No matter what happened, she would laugh and say "Man proposes and God disposes." Clearly I don't believe in that God who takes such a micro-interest in our doings. I do believe in taking responsibility for our lives, making plans and putting them in place, and then finding the flexibility necessary to meet our lives just as they are, no matter how we want them to be.

Losing the Self

Someone told me recently that a caregiver asked his mother whether she recognized him and she answered "I don't even recognize myself." She had dementia.

Before I worked in hospice, I'd tell people I thought I would die of cancer because of the way I watched my mom and other family members die, and then I'd shiver in fear. In America, cancer is the boogeyman. Now that I work in healthcare, I know there are several diseases that are worse, and the most common of those is the grindingly slow loss of personhood we call dementia. Someone with cancer or heart disease can usually still think and talk, interact and love right up to the end. People with dementia can't, but are caught in bodies that keep living long after their mind has been lost. And in hospice, about half of my patients come on to our service with that diagnosis.

Alzheimer's is the most common form of dementia, and the word itself has become a synonym for the disease. Dementia in itself is not fatal; unless the patient has "an event" - a stroke, a fall, or a heart attack — dementia itself brings death's release only when the brain forgets how to swallow even thickened water and baby food, and the patient starves to death. It's thought that this is a comfortable way to die, that the person who's bedbound and sleeping most of the day doesn't experience hunger in the same way a person who's up and moving around would. Still, it's hard for families to witness, and we have many discussions with people who are demanding we start I.V.s to inject water into their loved ones' arms and spoon food they can't swallow into their mouths.

Many people with dementia go through phases of agitation and anger, and it seems that most will eventually settle into sweetness and sleep. Social filters fall away, and perfectly nice people masturbate in public, smear their feces on the wall, and flick boogers at the nice chaplain. There was even an old nun who tried to bite me. Wandering is common, and the so-called memory units in the large chain care homes always seem to have people walking slowly through the hallways with puzzled expressions on their faces, or sitting by the door and asking when they can leave.

There are family members who are thrilled that a chaplain is visiting and ask me to read to the patient from the Bible, and I have a Gideon New Testament bristling with Post-Its for this purpose. Then there are times when I just sit silently, watching and thinking, wondering what I can do to help, wondering what there is for this person to teach me.

As a chaplain, I rely on words, and yet I have had to find a way to offer spiritual care to people who are mute, people who appear not to understand what I'm saying. I was taught in my residency to do an orientation, to call the patient by name, remind them who I am, tell them the date and say something about the time of year or the weather, and maybe talk about something I see in their room or something in the news. I always tell them that they're safe and if they're living in some sort of facility, I may explain that they're sick and they need the extra care.

If you are a person who has been directly affected by dementia, if you have cared for or witnessed someone you love go through this process, I'm sorry. I'm sorry for the pain dementia has caused you, and I also understand that the things I'm saying here may be hard for you to read. I'm not a doctor or a nurse, but I've provided care to hundreds of people in various stages of this loss of the self, and sat through countless hours of meetings where the disease was discussed. These things I'm saying come from that experience.

When I was a year or so into my work in hospice, just when I thought I knew what was going on, a family member taught me something important about visiting people with dementia. The patient was in her own home with a live-in caregiver. Her nearest relative was a nephew who was himself elderly. I phoned him after my visits and he was friendly and cheerful. Every few months, he drove to visit the patient and caregiver, to write checks and repair dripping faucets and chat. The caregiver was from the South Sea Islands. She lived in the front bedroom and her husband visited frequently. She'd redecorated the living room to her taste, with colorful fabric tossed on the dingy sofa and a grass mat over the carpet. She didn't have much to say to me, it seemed, but just opened the door and showed me to the back bedroom where the patient lived.

The patient was sweet. She was glad for company and answered my questions willingly. I looked around her room and commented on pictures, and she responded. She told me she'd worked outside of the home, she'd never had children, and her husband had a workshop back in the garage. She knew where the garage was.

One day I visited when her nephew was in town. He and the caregiver sat companionably in the living room while I went back to see the patient. When I emerged, I again said how sweet she was. I thought this was a compliment.

"No she isn't" he said. "I've told you this before." He began to get excited. He raised his voice, stood up and moved toward me to make his point. I stepped away from him until my back was to the wall.

"She was mean" her nephew said. "She was a mean woman." The caregiver sat on the couch, nodding her head, "umm-hmm"ing. He told me she'd treated her husband with contempt, so the man spent his days out in the garage drinking. She was mean to other family members, too — to his mother, for instance, who was the patient's sister. He said she might seem nice now that she had dementia, but she'd been relentlessly mean earlier in her life.

I left shaken, thinking they were the mean ones. I talked with co-workers about how he'd yelled at me, how nasty he and the caregiver were. But on reflection, I realized that while I'd thought I was praising him for being a part of a functional family, he wanted me to know that dealing with her hadn't been easy. He wanted credit for putting up with this woman, and they couldn't allow me to think it had always been peaches and cream. The patient and the nephew both taught me something about approaching patients with dementia.

Another time when I thought I knew what the patient needed, I made the stupid mistake of telling her daughter what I thought she should do. I reacted because I was disturbed by the patient. She lived in the memory unit of a good facility. She was one of the ones who paced endlessly, always with a worried look on her face. She picked at things. She seemed to see something on the carpet and would stop to bend over and scoop it up. Her pants were held up by suspenders to stop her from pulling them down and pooping in public. And the worst thing was, she cried. She cried all the time, sometimes streams of tears quietly running down her checks but sometimes sobbing, bent over with her head in her hands. It was awful. I immediately approached her, put my arm around her, and she leaned against my shoulder, crying, crying, crying.

I called her daughter after my first visit, and I raised the issue of depression. I told the daughter I thought something should be done to help the patient. Would she like our doctor to look at the patient's med list and see if she would prescribe an antidepressant for the old lady? The daughter really let me have it. This had been going on for months and months, and they had tried all of those drugs. Nothing helped. She visited her mother daily - did I think she hadn't noticed? Did I think it wasn't distressing to her? I was embarrassed and ashamed. I apologized, and made another note to myself to not think I could or should come charging in as if I could save the day.

Many months later I saw the mother and daughter sitting together and I joined them. The daughter held her mother's hand while we talked. The patient had moved into the next phase of her disease, and she had changed. She opened her eyes, closed her eyes, opened them again, and occasionally smiled. She had stopped crying. It was amazing. The daughter told me her mother's life story, told me their relationship hadn't always been easy but now she was glad she was able to visit daily, told me of other difficulties in her life, difficulties with her own health and her time spent with a friend who was also ill.

This woman had been so mad at me. Few family members have been so upset by my blundering. Now we sat and talked freely and it was such a pleasure. One of my ideas about my work is that I should just keep showing up so I'll be familiar and available when I'm needed; this conversation proved that sometimes that idea is the right one, but there's something else, too: keep showing up, and don't think you understand the patient better than their family does.

Maybe those of us who work with people with dementia are overwhelmed by our own inability to help. That's what I was trying to do with that lady, to come up with a solution to address my own discomfort with what I saw. But it's true, too, that sometimes some of us decide the patient is no longer a person and can be treated carelessly. It's most likely this will happen when a patient has been living for many months in a subsidized bed in a care facility. And the chances that a patient will be treated hastily, even neglected, are greater if no one visits them. This makes me think of a patient who was one of those, an elderly woman who was lost deep in dementia and alone. When we first met, she could say a few words. Now her eyes were blank and she repeated nonsense syllables, or, worse, seemed to be reporting on nightmares of danger and death. Who knows what her life experiences were, and what was lurking in those memory banks.

When she was still in her own apartment, before she was brought to the nursing home, there were some neighbors - we heard they were a part of a religious group - who had been watching out for her. She would sign checks and they would fill in the amount and send them to the landlord and the utility company. They told the social worker the son never visited, and they said they loved her and wanted to take care of her. We had a meeting with them and the son. He was a large man who had little to say except that he was in charge. Legally, he was right. We heard he emptied her apartment and paid her bills, and we never saw him or heard from him again. I left messages on his phone after I visited for a while and then gave up. Her neighbors visited for a while and I'd find her with lipstick kisses on her face but those visits stopped too.

The thing is, she didn't have any clothes. For months I'd only seen her wearing just one pair of pants, and they were too small. They looked like cotton hospital pajama bottoms that wrap around the waist, and since they were too small she sat parked in her wheelchair by the elevators with her diaper exposed. It didn't seem right. Several times I mentioned it to the facility's social worker, and each time she said she'd find something nicer for her. But each time I visited, she was still in the same too small pants with the exposed diaper.

Then it occurred to me I could do something about this. I went to Target, found some XXL pajama bottoms for $20, and took them to the patient. She was in bed and I gave them to an aide. The next time her name came up in our team meeting, I bragged about the new pants. Our home health aide said the patient didn't have any new pants. The next day, I went by and saw it was true.

I went to the social worker's office. "Where are the new pants?" was my greeting. She grudgingly walked back to the patient's room with me started to look in the closet.

She found all kinds of stuff, including two wall clocks and a half-eaten box of See's candy. A crowd of staff people gathered in the room, talking back and forth about where the pants were and who had put the clocks and candy there. I stood at the side, ignored and frustrated. None of this was getting us any closer to getting some decent clothes on the lady.

Finally I cried out "It's a dignity issue!" That was the magic word. The social worker rushed downstairs to the castoffs closet to find something and the crowd cleared. Now I had a moment to meet with the patient who had been sitting, bewildered, while all of this went on. We were settled, knee to knee, when a nurse and an aide came in talking loudly, grabbed her wheelchair, and rolled it away from me. "It's time to put her to bed" they said.

I could feel that I was about to lose my temper. From buying the pants to being there today while people ignored the patient and me and speculated about blame, it all felt like wasted time. I was rushing out through the lobby when a different social worker greeted me, and I brushed by her. I was so angry I didn't trust myself to speak. I went back to Target.

The next day, as I was entering through the lobby with my new bag of clothes, I saw the social worker. She hurried toward me.

"Ren, are you all right?"

"I'm so sorry…" I said,

"Oh we know all about it" she responded before I could go on. "That was so wrong. Really, it's a dignity issue!"

She said her boss, the head social worker, the head social worker, wanted to see me.

"Ren!" he said, "Thank you for taking care of your patients so well! It's a dignity issue!"

And so it continued, as I went to the memory unit. The words "dignity issue" were on everyone's lips. We held the new clothes against the patient's body to make sure they would fit, wrote her name on them with an indelible marker, charted them in inventory as hers, photographed them so if they were lost in the laundry they could be identified — in short, our patient's new pants were the event of the day.

She was in bed. I showed her the pants, a kind of rayon tie dye in turquoise blue, and she smiled. I showed her a nice button-front cotton shirt and she didn't even react. Then I showed her the t-shirt, a plain man's blue short sleeved crew neck from Target, and she cried out in joy. It really was a dignity issue.

Another patient who I was assigned around that same time had truly lost all dignity. When he was admitted to hospice, his paperwork had paragraphs detailing extreme family conflict among his kids – and then, there was a one line comment mentioning that he had tried to shoot himself. He was in a subsidized bed in a locked ward of a nursing home.

When I entered, people were parked in wheelchairs in the hall, some calling out, most silent. Their voices were background noise and got little response. Most of the staff people were in the dining room feeding patients who could no longer manage for themselves. I found the man I was coming to visit. He was in a wheelchair over in the corner, being fed by a young Chinese guy. I greeted the kid, who was glad to turn the patient over to me. I sat down and began to feed him myself, slowly and carefully.

He didn't meet my gaze, didn't respond to my words. His eyes were unfocused, looking somewhere in the middle distance. I couldn't tell whether this was caused by medication or despair or a combination of both. He did accept the mashed potatoes and puréed spinach as I spooned them into his mouth. At the next table, facility staffers were talking to each other while they fed patients. It sounded like India had sprung up behind my back while I wasn't looking - they spoke rapidly, loudly, in a language I didn't recognize, as if they were alone. One of the patients they were feeding had a problem with it and let out a roar from time to time. The attendants laughed and went on talking and spooning the food in. Between the noise they created and the noise the patients made, I begin to feel tense. I thought of how it was for my guy, old and sick and driven to a suicide attempt that landed him here where the noise is incessant and he's surrounded by strangers. Though he wasn't responding, I talked to him slowly, explaining where he was, explaining that he was here because he needed the help. If I were him, that's what I would want to know.

Suddenly he plunged his hand into the puréed spinach. I watched as he pulled his hand out and licked his fingers. He was feeding himself. I found the fellow who'd been caring for him staring into his cell phone in the hall, and turned the patient back over to him, glad to get away from the clamor and the despair in the dining room. I went to the nursing station to enter my chart notes. I exchanged greetings with a couple of staff members but no one had time to talk. When I washed my hands before I left, I saw a used band-aid sitting by the sink.

I walked out feeling sad for us all. For the patients who are stuck in this place against their will, either roaring in protest or silently staring into space; for the staff members who are overworked and underpaid and perhaps have had to develop defenses against the suffering they witness for eight hours a day every day; and for the chaplain who is powerless to help. I remembered my early recognition that my presence can remind people, including staff, that there's a spiritual element to this passage between birth and death, and hoped that maybe I brought something like that to that difficult place on that day.

With another patient, a woman in her 80s whose loving family had put her in a nice apartment in an expensive facility, a place where the fees were high enough that it was more adequately staffed, the help I offered was a little more practical. The staff started her day by bringing her pills, then they cleaned and dressed her, and left her in front of the television. They checked on her several times a day and her door was kept open so they could glance in when they walked down the hall. Someone took her to the dining room for meals.

She was confused. She forgot she couldn't walk and after one visit I stood in the hall and watched as she bounced up and down, trying to get out of her wheelchair. I was relieved to see her abandon the effort; if she'd been able to stand, the chances were that she'd fall. Once we were sitting in front of the television together when she said "I found this thing. What is it?" and lifted her shirt to show me her fingers grasping the nipple on her sagging breast. "Nothing to worry about" I assured her.

There was a visit when I entered the room and didn't see her in the living room or the bedroom alcove and then looked in the open bathroom door and saw her sitting on the toilet, nude, while an attendant vigorously scrubbed her face with a washcloth. The smell told me that she was having a bowel movement. I told the attendant I'd come back later. I liked her and I didn't want to see her like that, powerless and treated more like a thing than a person. If I had the authority to speak to the aide, I'm sure she'd say that the patient didn't know the difference, that the boss said she can only spend so much time in each apartment, that they've always done it this way. But sitting naked on a toilet and having a bowel movement while someone scrubs your face when you're already confused – I just kept coming back to how hard it looked.

When her decline began, the aides stopped getting her out of bed during the day and began putting a nasal cannula - the plastic device that wraps around the ears and delivers oxygen to the nose through two little prongs - on her. She ripped it off. I found it on the floor and told her it could keep her more comfortable, and she said she hated it and she wanted it off. Our doctor said a small fan pointed toward the patient's face would help, so I bought one and installed it by her bed. My patient was very happy about it. I spoke to the aide who was caring for her that day, told her the fan was doctors' orders, and she said she'd keep the cannula off and the fan on.

Later that week I came back to see her. The fan was on top of the dresser, unplugged. The oxygen concentrator was pumping, but the nasal cannula was back on the floor. From her bed, she gestured toward "That white thing."

"That's a fan," I said, "and actually I bought it for you."

"No, you didn't," she replied. "My friend did."

I was glad she remembered I was her friend, even if she didn't recognize me in that moment. I plugged the fan in and turned it toward her face.

When her decline shifted into actively dying, the stage where the patient stops eating and starts sleeping around the clock, when the breathing becomes rapid and shallow and the hands and feet go cold, I went to see her every day. She was in bed, she was unresponsive, and the cannula was in place. Even if I found someone and invoked the hospice doctor's authority and got them to take the cannula off, another aide would be on duty in a few hours, and she would put it back on, as she was trained to do. I hoped my lady wasn't too bothered by it now. At least she had family who visited and staff who checked on her.

In a similar assisted-living facility, I visited a man with dementia who had lived there for years. The things in his room — the pictures on the walls, the furniture, the books — indicated that he had been someone who cared about art, someone who sought out beauty. He had been a doctor, he had never married, he had no family, and now he was alone. His disease was so advanced that the facility staff no longer put him in his wheelchair to go to the dining room, but sat at his side feeding him baby food while he stayed in bed.

As I browsed around his room on my first visit, looking for clues about him, I noticed he had two copies of Rilke's *Selected Poems*. I picked one up and said out loud that, in an amazing coincidence, I also had two copies of the same book. He didn't respond. I opened it, and found my favorite poem — the one that starts "You see, I want a lot" — and read it aloud. He'd used folded bits of Kleenex as bookmarks; I turned to the pages where they lay and read those poems as well. He lay on his bed, listening, blinking his eyes, not moving.

There was a strong smell of urine, so strong that it lingered in my nose after I left his room. Thinking it was coming from a wet diaper, I spoke to someone at the nurses' station about it. She frowned and barked, "I'll get that carpet cleaned again." I try to advocate for my patients without irritating people, so I thanked her and left. The smell remained as I continued my visits.

Each time I went, I'd look through his books for something to read. There was more Rilke. Once it was *archy and mehitabel*, Don Marquis's free-verse stories of a cockroach and a cat written in the 1930s; another time it was Paul Tillich, the twentieth-century Christian philosopher. These were his books, this was his taste.

One day I entered and found my patient in bed as usual, but slumped against the wall with a blanket pulled over his head. I looked closely to see whether he was breathing. He was, and so I put my hand on his shoulder, said I hoped he was comfortable, and told him I thought I'd keep reading to him.

I started with more Tillich, but on that day it seemed too heavy, and so I returned to *archy and mehitabel*. The free verse was challenging: it required a delicate pause at the end of each line, and the mildly archaic language threw up words I don't often use. Still, I was enjoying it. I might have even been showboating a little.

I stopped when an aide came in and greeted the patient loudly. She pulled the blanket off his head; he looked at her. She asked him if he wanted anything, and he said, "Drink."

She gave him some Ensure, and he gulped it down. She left. The patient looked at me. I explained again who I was, showed him the book we'd been reading. He blinked and tugged at the blanket. I asked whether he was cold — the window was open, perhaps because of the smell in the room — and when he nodded, I continued to talk as I reached to pull up the warm blanket that was folded at the foot of the bed. Suddenly he spoke:

"I can't hear a word you're saying."

I had been reading to myself.

Shouting information slowly at someone is different from reading free verse in a comforting voice. I really can't shout *archy and mehitabel*. Maybe I could manage to shout one Rilke poem. But I was out of time anyway, so that visit was over.

I spoke to the head of the unit about the urine smell again. She said it was probably in the mattress and thus it was my company's responsibility. Again I didn't argue, but called the man in my office who handles these things.

On my next visit, weeks later, my patient was awake, he could speak short sentences, and the smell of urine was gone from the room. It was like a miracle.

I pulled up a chair and reminded him who I was and told him we'd been visiting for a while. He listened and nodded. I doubt he remembered me, but what I was saying was okay with him. I asked him whether he was comfortable — comfort is the goal in hospice, and this question is required. Then I asked, as I have wanted to ask a patient with dementia so many times,

"Is this life okay with you?"

He looked at me, puzzled.

"I can see you've been an active man. I heard you were a doctor and you've helped many people. Now you're sick and you need help and you have to stay in bed. Is that okay?"

"Yes!" he answered. "It's nice!"

There was an old radio on the table next to his bed, tuned to the jazz station. The reception was always slightly off and I found the static irritating. "And do you like the music?" I asked.

"Oh, yes!" he answered.

I don't know why he could hear me one day and not another. I don't know how it is to be bedridden, in diapers, sleeping most of the day and dependent on a stranger for a glass of Ensure. To me — able to stand and walk away, to start my car and drive to my next visit — it looked like tor-ment. To him, on that day, it was apparently just life.

He never spoke again. When I arrived and saw that the caregivers had changed his radio to hip-hop, I changed it back to the jazz station. And I kept reading to him, just in case. His decline was slow until suddenly he was transition-ing and then I received an email that he had died in the night. I hope he was really and truly not bothered by the way dementia had taken away what I think of as a life.

There was a woman who I visited for many months who had a bed in a large sort of women's dorm room in a skilled nursing facility. It never looked to me as if she had much of a life, and yet she woke every day and opened her mouth willingly, even eagerly, for the aide to spoon in the baby food that sustained her. The room had a big old fash-ioned television that roared out soap operas. It drove me crazy. One or two of the patients watched or listened, and the rest slept. My patient slept. She hadn't spoken in years. Her husband had died, and the friend who was listed as decision maker on her information sheet was too old and sick to visit. I was it, and I visited as often as possible. I brought her stuffed animals to hold.

Sometimes, she would scream. I mean, just scream. I was visiting one day when she began and the woman in the bed next to her screamed back and I tried to soothe my pa-tient while the two of them shared their feelings this way until finally I could only put my forehead on the bed railing and cry in frustration and sorrow. That's what I mean when I say that I wonder whether the patient's life is worth living. But she kept eating and she didn't lose weight and our nurse couldn't enter any signs of decline in her chart, so we discharged her. I still looked in when I was visiting other patients in that nursing home but couldn't spend much time with her. I learned that she died from one of the aides.

I had a different patient in another of those basic skilled nursing facilities who screamed a lot. Before she was on our service, when I was visiting my patients, I would hear her down the hall:

"Oh my God

"Let me go / there he goes

"They're coming up again

"I'm lonely"

When she came on our service, our doctor adjusted her medications and she screamed less. But when she spoke, screaming or whispering, it was always about being lonely, about wanting to die. Family visited her regularly and her walls were covered with photographs – but she wanted her life to end. Except it didn't.

It was easy for me to agree that her life was going on longer than was reasonable. Her family members, one daughter in law in particular, would drive long distances to visit her and they all seemed to want her to keep living. Since I didn't see any pleasure in the life she had and thought her screams and pleas meant she didn't either, I'd ask her whether she was afraid to die. "Yes" she'd whisper. And so, since she had been a church-goer back when she could still walk, and since the family members who visited her were very religious, I'd talk about trusting God, about remembering that God offered the ultimate safety. She was so old and so small; when I talked, she'd open her eyes and look at me as if she was trying to figure out whether I was telling the truth.

She lived on and on. We talked about her incessantly in our team meetings. Was she eating less? Sleeping more? Losing weight? She started at such a low point, already bed bound for a couple of years, eating little bites of pureed food, not really able to respond to a question, it was hard to describe her as declining. Yet we did, many times, until we couldn't, and then we would discharge her for extended prognosis – the Medicare term that means she's too healthy for hospice -- and then, months later, something would happen and she'd come back on our service.

I went through months where I didn't visit, because I didn't feel there was anything I could do for her. And then her hospice nurse would say the old lady was lonely and ask me to see her, so I'd go back and she'd be responsive and I'd feel useful so I'd pick up the visits again.

She had many episodes of aspiration pneumonia, caused when the patient inhales food into the lungs. Pneumonia used to be called "the old person's friend": it can be treated with antibiotics, or it can be the mechanism that releases the patient from this life. I asked her nurse whether she'd talked with the family about it before she started the drugs. She said they'd agreed to the antibiotics when she called them. She said the patient deserved them.

Then, during a time when she was off of our service, she died. We heard that one night, with nothing special going on, she went to sleep and didn't wake up. I hope I was telling her the truth and that she's safe now, wherever she is, and I deeply hope she's no longer calling out "Oh my God – Let me go – I'm lonely." I hope she's found her self again.

Bringing Death

I've been helping people end their lives since my first months working as a hospice chaplain. It hasn't been easy.

I've mentioned the grief and confusion I felt when I was a brand-new chaplain in Oregon and one of my patients used their Death with Dignity law to end her life. Six years later, I was back in California when its law – called the End of Life Option Act and referred to as EOLOA – was passed. Some hospices told employees to not even talk about it. The small community non-profit I was a part of intended to participate fully, even enthusiastically, and scheduled many workshops to teach us how the law had worked for the last ten years in Oregon and what we should be prepared for. The surprise was that people weren't using the law because of physical pain. They were using it because their lives had lost meaning and dignity. They were using it because they were worried about money. They were using it because they'd lost control of their lives.

I was one of two people in the company who had experienced physician-aided suicide, and I settled into my comfortable position of being an old pro. We were told our participation was voluntary. I was in. The workshops talked about how to obey the law medically, but I learned that nothing could prepare me emotionally.

Here's what we were taught: The patient has to have a terminal illness and a life expectancy of less than six months, and they have to have the mental competency to ask for the drugs, acknowledge they understand that they will cause their death, and hold the glass containing them and drink its contents without help. There's a two week waiting period after the first request, and two doctors have to sign off on the patient's decision. This is all good, since it means no one can hide behind the law to end anyone else's life. We also learned the drugs are expensive, and Medicare doesn't pay for them.

The manager of the spiritual care department told us we had a patient who wanted to use EOLOA as soon as it came into effect. The patient had never had a chaplain visit, and it was thought he should get one on his team now – particularly because he had a daughter who was objecting to his ending his life, apparently because of her religious beliefs. The other two chaplains looked at our manager with furrowed brows as she explained the case, and I raised my hand to volunteer.

He was a man in his 80's who had been in a facility for five years, When he'd first moved there, he'd been able to use a wheelchair to go to the dining room for meals and bingo. Now he was bedridden. When I went to meet him, he was very open to me, warm and straightforward, kind of charming even as he lay on a hospital bed wearing nothing but a diaper. I offered to cover his massive bare chest and legs with a sheet but he refused. I kept my eyes on his face.

We talked about his life and his family. He'd been a part of the wave of military men who settled in the bay area after the war. He'd had the sort of solid blue collar life that was available then: acquiring a trade, moving up in a company, marrying his sweetheart, buying a house, and starting a family. He'd retired happily only a few years before his heart began to fail and he ended up here.

He told me about the gradual erosion of his dignity that he could no longer bear, that he didn't want to lie in bed with a wet diaper calling out to aides who walked by his door, ignoring him and his call light. He worried about draining the family's resources and leaving his wife poor and alone. He was bored and humiliated. He was done. His wife and the two grown children who lived locally agreed with him, but the daughter who lived at a distance was fighting his decision.

My company's doctor called a team meeting the day before he was scheduled to take the drugs and the distant daughter was mentioned. Faces turned in my direction. I agreed to call her. She was angry and insisted her father shouldn't die this way. It turned out she was only a few hours away, and we set up a time to meet in the nursing home that afternoon.

Many people from our company and the facility showed up for that meeting. The daughter got everyone's attention as she demanded to know whose fault it was that his health had deteriorated to this point, why he was no longer going to the dining room for meals or the activities room for bingo, why no one had found musical groups that would come and sing to him. She insisted we try everything to make his life worth living, so a dusty Hoyer lift was brought in to move him from his bed to a wheelchair and suddenly his tiny room was packed full of chattering pastel-clad aides getting a training in using it and he was swinging through the air, clutching the straps and shouting. It was bizarre. At one point the daughter and I were off to the side together and I asked her quietly if she was a part of a religion that forbade suicide. She was startled. She wasn't religious at all. She just didn't want her father to die.

Suddenly he shouted

"No! Enough! I'm through talking about this! My mind's made up - I'm going to die tomorrow!"

He was in the wheelchair. The facility staff ladies scattered and it was just him, his hospice nurse, me, and his daughter. It was startling to see how completely she gave in to him. I had no doubt I was watching the two of them go through a dance they'd practiced for decades, that she had played her part when she had tried to change his mind, he'd played his when he demanded that she do it his way, and now she was satisfied. The nurse and I turned to go and he called me back for a goodbye kiss.

I was in our weekly meeting the next day when I saw the message that he was dead. I was surprised by the tears that ran down my cheeks. As we went through the litany of deaths, the stories of the new admissions, and reviewed patients to be sure they were still hospice appropriate, I turned over my patient's death and my reaction in my mind. When the meeting ended, I turned to the doctor sitting next to me and asked,

"Should we be doing this? We just helped someone commit suicide. It would be easier if he had visible physical suffering, but his suffering was hidden from us. His suffering was the loss of control over his own life and the loss of purpose in living."

I felt his powerlessness. I also felt the many suicides I've experienced in my life rustle in their sleep.

"What's the difference between what we did today and my cousin Jon going into the woods with a shotgun and blowing his head off? Aren't we just sanitizing the same act?"

He said maybe we were, that in each case the person was experiencing suffering so extreme they could no longer live, and that in one case they did it with our help and in the other they did it alone. That was the word I needed. What if, for instance, my cousin had had two doctors, a nurse, a social worker and a chaplain to talk to about his despair? Wasn't his isolation at least partly the cause of his sad suicide? So, I saw, we can bring dignity to our people.

The doctor told me about an early patient of his who was looking at a long slow decline, in physical pain, with increasing dependence on his elderly wife, who shot himself. He had to do it alone. So Death with Dignity, or the End of Life Option Act, or Physician-Assisted Suicide can do better than that. We can do better than that, even if it's hard.

I began to take all of the EOLOA cases. We weren't allowed to bring it up - the patient had to mention it first - but I was called in to explain the law to groups of weeping family members. I pointed out that choosing the day and time meant they would be present when the patient took their last breath, and that the patient would be able to take back the control they'd lost when their health began to fail. I talked about dignity. I talked about love. Usually, I followed up with family members after a death, but I wasn't present when the death occurred.

Then, a woman who I'd been visiting for months decided to use the Act, and she asked me to be present. When we first met, she was living in her daughter's house, and she could get around using her walker. She was satisfied with her life. She couldn't go out any more, but a few old friends came to visit. Gradually she grew weaker until moving from her bed to the easy chair at its side became an issue. Her daughter thought her mother should try harder and urged her to do exercises, to build her strength back up, to free herself of diapers and dependence. I watched while she and her daughter erupted in screaming fights. She began to describe her life as "misery" and she wanted to end it. My company still forbade us from telling patients about EOLOA, and it was hard to hear her say repeatedly that she wished there were a way to end her life, know there was one, and remain silent. But she found out, and asked to start the process. She and her daughter began a struggle over her choice that lasted months while the doctor, the nurse, and I talked to each of them. She won.

The night before she was scheduled to take the lethal drugs, they had a family dinner. Everyone came. After the meal was finished, they came into her room to say goodbye to her, one at a time. When the doctor and the nurse and I arrived the next morning, everyone was ready. She asked me to help the nurse prepare the drugs – in those days we used a pile of Seconal capsules that had to be opened and emptied by hand. The nurse and I worked together at the kitchen table while the doctor sat next to us completing the paperwork. It was surreal and sacred.

After the meds were mixed, I whispered into the patient's ear, asking if she wanted a prayer. She was the kind of Christian who knows she's going to heaven, and was looking forward to seeing dead friends when she got there.

"You can pray for me after I'm gone" was her answer.

She fell asleep within minutes after she took the drugs, and I was sitting so close to her I could see the change in her face as death arrived. The doctor remained quiet and steady, watching her pulse as she slept deeply and then, after 20 minutes, he declared her dead. The doctor and nurse left the room and I stayed with the family to follow her request and ask her children to join hands and say the Lord's Prayer with me.

She had as much life as she wanted, and she said good-bye gracefully. She was good preparation for my next EOLOA case, also a mother, but one without the financial resources to get the drugs that acted so quickly. I was surprised when I made my initial visit and learned she had initiated the End of Life Option Act 12 days earlier. It was Friday and she planned to take the drugs on Monday.

She'd been in a big senior facility for years, going downstairs with the help of her walker to activities and meals, making friends among other mobile old people, and occasionally going out to dinner with her family. Her daughter lived half an hour away but visited often, her son a little less so.

She'd been diagnosed with cancer just a few months earlier. It was moving fast: her skin was already turning yellow and she could no longer walk. But she was awake and alert and clear, and she still had her sense of humor. She said she just wanted to skip the helplessness and pain that she saw in her future. I admired how calm she was about it. The date of her death was circled on her calendar, and for her it couldn't come soon enough.

Her daughter was there, and she and I moved to an open area with sofas and chairs outside of the apartment and talked for about an hour. She was crying before the door closed; the patient's decision wasn't so clear for her, partly because she was a devout Catholic and she was afraid for her mother's eternal soul. I couldn't tell her about that, beyond suggesting she trust the priest who'd said EOLOA wasn't a sin, but I was able to explain how it was likely to go – the team would arrive and give her mother the lethal drugs, and then her mother would go to sleep and eventually stop breathing. And I could say that in every case our patient had died peacefully. They were the last visit of my work week, and I parted from the two of them with smiles and hugs.

Two days later, I saw on the weekend report that the patient had had a terrible episode of delirium the night before. She'd started screaming and locked herself in her bathroom, not knowing who or where she was. Someone from the facility got the door open, and someone from my company had given her drugs that had calmed her.

I usually fiddle around on my first day back at work, reading emails and planning my visits, but on that day I immediately put on my shoes and lipstick and drove to see her. The EOLOA law requires mental competence, and if delirium continued to grip her mind, she wouldn't be eligible to use the drugs.

Her small apartment was filled with her children, her adult grandchildren, and the grandchildren's' spouses. As I moved toward her and held out my hand, she said

"I don't remember your name, but I do remember that pretty face." I asked her whether she still wanted to end her life and she said she did.

"I've had a good life" she said and once again told me she didn't want to continue living with pain and loss of independence.

These few days had given her daughter time to accept her mother's choice, and the episode of delirium had perhaps given her an indication of what might be in her mother's future. She was calm. The patient and her daughter said the two week waiting period was over and she'd like to take the EOLOA drugs that very day, and asked if the doctor and nurse could come, and if I could be with them.

I called my coworkers and told them what was going on. Both agreed to come that afternoon.

I suggested to the family that we calm down the energy in the room to save the patient's strength, and the grandchildren moved out to the open area outside of the apartment. I asked the patient if she'd like to take a nap, and she closed her eyes and plunged into a deep sleep. Her son and daughter and I moved through the apartment, tidying up, getting everything arranged. The daughter was tearful, the son anxious. The patient had asked for the less expensive drugs, and they required a 40 minute drive to a special pharmacy that would put the formula together, so the daughter's husband set out to pick them up. It was moving fast.

I left, took a walk, had a turkey sandwich, and calmed myself. When I returned the patient was still asleep. I stroked her arm and said her name. She didn't respond. I tried again, louder. Nothing. Earlier we'd been worried about her being lost in delirium. Now my worry was we wouldn't be able to wake her.

When the doctor arrived, he went down on one knee and said her name softly and she woke instantly. She smiled at him and he at her. Doctors are powerful.

"We're all here to help you with the end of life option you've chosen. Is it still what you want to do?"

"Yes!" she said clearly.

He went to the table and got the medicine and walked back. "I have the medicine here. Do you understand what will happen if you drink it?"

"Yes!" she said loudly. "I'll die!" She smiled. I moved to her daughter and put my arm around her. Her body leaned into mine. Her brother stood alone, turned in on himself. The patient, this sick old lady in her 90's, took the glass from the doctor in both hands, held it to her mouth and drank it down. She tipped her head back to drain out every drop, smacked her lips and beamed at us. A collective "Wow" went through the room.

After that, her children hugged her and kissed her and told her they loved her as she fell asleep. Then the five of us sat and looked at her. And looked. And looked. I thought I should be doing something and wondered what it was, and remembered that early ICU visit when I understood it was my job to be the visual reminder that there is a spiritual side to death. So I sat, silent, and let that be enough.

And we waited.

The expensive drugs act quickly, and they're the ones we have the most experience with. These drugs were working slowly. After an hour had passed, we began to talk quietly. After two hours, I saw the doctor and nurse exchanging worried glances and heard the doctor ask quietly whether there were other drugs in the apartment in case he needed to add them to the mix.

I suggested to the son and daughter that we go for a walk and "break up the energy." They both leapt up in agreement. We left, pausing to talk with their children who were still sitting outside, waiting. They'd been drinking up their grandmother's Scotch and were relaxed and laughing, but they quieted when they saw us. None of them wanted to join us.

The nearness of death had us in a sort of bubble, a time apart from the regular ticking of clocks and worries about getting and spending. At these times, life can become delicious. The trees and sky looked beautiful. Cars passed and I thought they couldn't know how near death was. The three of us walked past tidy suburban houses and I said we never know what's going on behind closed doors. The patient's daughter agreed, said she was having the same thought. We walked for 15 or 20 minutes, mostly remaining silent, and then returned to the apartment. When we came back inside, everything was the same.

She died after four hours. The doctor didn't need to use any more drugs. She was never uncomfortable, just asleep. I went to tell the grandkids and they came inside the apartment to gather around her body; they and her children displayed the mix of sorrow and relief that usually accompanies a good death.

I was glad to have been a part of it, to feel useful, to give the patient what she most wanted and to support her family. I knew her for less than a week and then she was gone. Her daughter called me once in a while after that to talk about her mother's death, and to cry and tell me how grateful she was to my company.

But not everyone in my hospice agreed with this practice of bringing death. One of our doctors was furious when I talked to his patient about the option.

The patient was the husband, and he and his wife were both at the end of long careers as academics. Their children were grown and launched into the world, and they had been looking forward to an active retirement when the husband was diagnosed with cancer. He worked for as long as he could, and when he came on hospice he was already using heavy drugs to control his pain. He sat in a wheelchair and dozed off and on while I talked with his wife and then he woke and raised his head and whispered that he was afraid of what was to come. I asked what he was afraid of, and he whispered one word: pain. My company's guidelines had changed and I was allowed to tell patients about EOLOA, so I asked if they'd heard about it. The patient's wife said she'd read something when it came into law, but they didn't know the specifics. I outlined the procedure that would allow him to make an exit before the pain became unbearable, and they asked if they could start the process immediately. I knew he didn't have much time left, so I finished the visit and called their doctor from my car. He wasn't working, so I called the doctor who was on duty. He came to the house that evening and started the two week waiting period.

A few days later, their original doctor called me in to the office. We'd been friends when I started at the company - I'd even thought he was flirting with me for a while - but this was not friendly. His face was already red when he entered the room, and he began yelling before he sat down. I've heard it before from doctors: Who do you think you are?! How dare you talk to my patients without my permission?! He said he was late because he'd been filing a complaint with the boss. It was hard. I wasn't afraid for my job; I just don't do well with people shouting at me.

When I visited the family later that week, the patient's wife was crying as she told me the doctor had been there. He had said that it would be a failure if the patient used drugs to end his life, and had urged the dying man to be strong and endure a natural death to set a good example for the children. I believe the phrase "be a hero" was used. Both the patient and his wife were distressed and there wasn't much I could say. He died a handful of days after that visit, too soon to access the drugs that would have ended his suffering. I don't think that doctor ever forgave me, but I still felt I'd done the right thing for the patient.

Many months after that, I was asked to take part in an EOLOA that was started in plenty of time, but on the day our patient took the drugs, it felt like something went wrong.

He was one of those people everyone loved. He was sweet and undemanding and, although he was in his 60's, there was an innocence about him. That makes the story of his death particularly hard to tell.

He lived with his aged cat in a large building downtown, and when I rang the bell by his name on the directory, he called out that his apartment was unlocked. When I walked in, I saw that it would have been hard for him to get up to open the door for me: one of his legs was propped up on the bed, grotesquely swollen by the tumor that would end his life. It was hard to see how he could get around and take care of himself, but he had to. He was alone.

Although our nurse had been visiting him for a couple of months, he hadn't wanted to see a chaplain. Then, a week earlier, he had told his nurse he thought it was time for us to help him die, and she had called me. Now he was eager to talk.

He said a suspicious lump had appeared on his arm less than a year earlier; the doctors looked at it, told him it was cancer, and gave him radiation treatments. He said there was another lump in his leg, and he kept asking the doctors to look at it. They did, but he didn't think they really paid attention to it. When it became so large that his leg began to swell, he went back to the clinic and they looked more closely and agreed with him that it was also cancer. They said there was no treatment available and recommended he go on hospice. He didn't trust those doctors any more and was glad to switch over to our care. He was very clear about every detail of this story.

He said he'd had a good life: he had friends and had always had a place to live and enough to eat. He hadn't married and didn't have children, but this didn't bother him. Although he hadn't been much of a churchgoer, he believed in God and in heaven. We talked about quality of life and agreed that he still had it. He could go out with his walker every day and sit on a park bench or in a Starbucks and talk to people. He liked to read, and he watched a few television shows. He was content and he wanted to keep living this way as long as possible. The question was, how long that would be. The issue was pain. He'd been through enough already to know how bad it could get, and he didn't want to stick around if it got worse.

"So then," he said, "When it gets bad, I'll just force myself to chug down the medicine and I'll die."

"Wait!" I interrupted. "Maybe we can take a look at that. Maybe instead of 'forcing yourself to chug it down,' you can see it as a gift you're giving yourself."

He liked that, thought it over, and smiled.

Looking back at it, maybe I shouldn't have interrupted him. Maybe I should have talked less and listened more. But in that first meeting, I went on to explain the process. He nodded as I listed the first conversation with the doctor, the two week waiting period, the necessity that he be able to take the drugs without help. When my explanation came to the cost, he broke in. This was the first he'd heard that Medicare didn't cover the drugs. I emailed the social worker while he watched, asking her to investigate. She answered later to say he would have to find the money himself, and that the least expensive drugs cost hundreds of dollars.

Weeks passed. I visited often, and asked him every time whether he was sure an assisted death was what he wanted. Each time, he said he was. He said he didn't want to die, but repeated he didn't want to live in pain; and he was worried that the disease would progress until he missed the window and would be unable to take the medicine. I promised him we'd take care of him if that happened. I told him that hospice doctors are better at pain control than regular doctors, but said I understood his fears. In the back of my mind I knew if he became unable to care for himself there wouldn't be enough help for him alone in his little apartment, and the options, the places he might be moved to that offered subsidized care when he needed diapers and heavy drugs, wouldn't be pleasant. But I didn't mention this; he was already frightened enough.

One of his friends flew in from out of state to visit when she heard he was on hospice, and another friend visited on weekends. One day he told me he'd had trouble getting in and out of his friend's car because his leg was so swollen and weak. He and his friend had to "lift the leg as if it was a piece of wood." He couldn't go outside alone with his walker any more, either. He was stuck inside and he was full of fear, imagining the tumor growing inside of him. He thought this was the sign he'd been waiting for, and said it was time to die.

There was a sudden flurry of emails, and the next thing I knew, he'd moved into a hospice house. When I visited I found him sitting in the living room, smiling and chatting with the staff and anyone else who happened by. His Social Security check was coming in a day or two, and, instead of paying the rent on his apartment, he'd use that money for the lethal drugs. He'd arranged with friends to be with him when he died and asked me to join them, but instead we had to say goodbye that day: I was going on retreat for a week, so this would be our last meeting.

I thought about him while I meditated in silence on the day of his death. I was sorry I couldn't be with him.

When I came home, though, I learned he'd changed his mind. The doctor, the nurse, and his friends had been at his bedside, the lethal drugs were prepared, and this quiet undemanding man held up his hand and said "Stop!" He liked living in the hospice house and wanted to enjoy it for as long as he could. Hospice houses are expensive, but no one said a word to him about money. He lived there for another week.

The second time he was scheduled to die, I sat with him. A volunteer who he'd become close to arrived and set up a little music system to play the songs he'd asked for. They started with "Amazing Grace" and then ranged from Wagner to Cole Porter. He was quiet, settled, and determined. The doctor and nurse came into the room with the medicine, and the doctor held up the glass.

"Do you understand what this is for?"

"Yes. It will make me die. I'm ready." He took the glass and drank it. Only then did he turn to me and ask me to call his friends. I agreed. The music played. The volunteer wept.

Then something horrible happened. He jerked upright; his arm shot into the air and he screamed as if a bolt of lightning had run through his body. The doctor and I looked at each other in shock. I thought of the volunteer and didn't want to scare him, so I remained silent while I wondered, Was it physical pain? Had he changed his mind again, now that it was too late? Did he regret what we had helped him do? Had he just seen death?

His head fell back on the pillow and he closed his eyes. He fell asleep and didn't wake again; he remained still for hours, sometimes snoring softly, while the volunteer and I sat by his side.

When the volunteer said he had to leave, I asked him to wait while I phoned the patient's friends and tell them he was dying. Out of the room, I found the doctor and we talked. I asked him what had happened when the patient had jumped up and screamed. He said he didn't know. He reminded me that the drugs we use are always changing, dependent on the patient's finances and what's available from the drug companies. He put out a call for a fresh volunteer to come and stay with the patient. We were all exhausted.

Later that night, I got a message telling me the patient had died. A volunteer and a hospice house aide had been by his side and his last breath had been a peaceful one.

He died the way he wanted to because he was afraid of pain and helplessness. He died when he did because he had to choose between paying rent or buying the drugs that would end his life. He lived for a week past the date circled on the calendar because the hospice house could be generous and allow him to, but he couldn't afford to live in his apartment with his cat for another week or another month. He slept for so long between taking the drugs and dying because the drugs he was able to afford were less efficient than the ones available to wealthier people.

EOLOA gave him back the control over his life that cancer had taken from him, but it was money and the lack of it that determined the hour of his death.

Ritual Helps

When I first worked for the large for-profit hospice, all social workers and chaplains were assigned regular on-call shifts on nights and weekends. We had several hundred patients and covered a large geographic area, so it wasn't unusual for me to be summoned to get up, get dressed, and drive for 30 or 40 minutes to meet some strangers who were having one of the worst nights of their lives. I approached each of these visits with my heart in my throat, and almost always walked back to my car smiling with relief and gratitude.

Initially, that hospice required chaplains and social workers to examine the patient and make the official death pronouncement. I raised my hand in every monthly meeting to say I wasn't qualified to do this and shouldn't be asked to. I finally got the big boss to agree but, before that policy was made official, I was called again to a room full of people gathered around a corpse who were waiting for a nurse but got me instead. I couldn't tell them about the new policy and refuse to do what was needed, so I stepped forward and laid my fingers on the neck of the body while they watched, then stood up and told them he was dead. I was relieved when he didn't start breathing again and prove me wrong. After that, I could sit with his daughters and hear the story of his life and hand them Kleenex while they cried. We could hold hands and say a prayer over his body, and I could let them know when they had done enough and it was time to leave.

But not everyone who dies has a family. I learned this on one of my first on-call shifts in hospice. Death visits had been covered in orientation, but, though it was nearly midnight when my phone rang and a nice lady in a call center gave me the name of the man who had died and the address of the facility he was in, I called my boss to ask her to tell me again what I was supposed to do. I was nervous, and I wanted to get it right. I woke her, but she was nice about it. She told me to comfort family members who were there or find their names and numbers in the patient's chart and phone them if they weren't, call the mortuary to pick up the body, and complete the paperwork.

It was a long drive. After I found the nursing home, and then the nurse who'd called in the death, I asked whether family was present. She told me the patient was alone — in fact, he had been there for three years and had never had a visitor. She told me she'd already called the mortuary. She was going through my checklist for me, and I realized that really, I was there just to collect a signature and close his file. But it seemed I should do something, so I asked to see him.

He was in the middle bed in a three-bed room. The curtains on either side were drawn for privacy. I found a chair and sat inside the fabric cave with his dead body. A television murmured from one side, a guy snored on the other. I touched the corpse, blessed it, talked to it, told him he wasn't alone. For his sake, and mine, and the staff's, we had a visit. I waited with him until the undertaker came and walked with the two of them, the man who picks up dead bodies in the middle of the night and the man who had died alone, to the van that was parked outside. It was a beautiful night and the undertaker and I commented on it and smiled when we parted. For a short time, I was the patient's family. I hoped he knew I was there. The nurse did, and she called out a "Thank you!" when I left.

Many months later, after I'd gotten used to going out at night when someone died, I had one of my favorite death visits. It was to a Vietnamese family in a nursing home. This time, it was early enough in the evening that there were still several women at the facility's nursing station when I arrived, and they laughed when one of them told me the family had been waiting for me -- according to their religion, I was "the death lady," and I was the only one allowed to touch the corpse. When I entered the patient's room I saw a body lying in bed, wearing an oxygen mask attached to a machine that was still pumping air into his dead lungs. His wife and two grown children sat huddled in the bit of space at the foot of the bed. The curtain was drawn between the patient and his roommate, but the tableau was open to anyone walking down the hall.

I greeted the family, put on gloves, turned off the noisy machine and removed the mask. He was a small old

Vietnamese man. The wife, who spoke no English, handed me his false teeth and gestured toward the body. Her daughter spoke: "She wants you to put them in." I tried not to show my discomfort as I took the teeth and turned toward the dead man. His lips were stiff, and I struggled while the family watched. After I managed to get the lower plate in, I turned to ask the daughter if that wasn't enough. She translated and her mother said no and gestured with impatience, so I turned back and put the uppers in too, relieved that they went into his mouth more easily. I turned back to the family. The wife gave me a tiny piece of gold — it was the backing piece to an earring — and gestured to the dead man's mouth. Put it in? Yes, put it in. This, the daughter said, was so he'd be wealthy in his next life. Placing it on his tongue was so much easier than inserting the teeth that I could relax and move slowly to make this a ritual - I could be "the death lady" for the family. The final offering was a shiny penny, clearly payment for the ferryman. After it was in place, I turned to see what was to be done next, and was almost disappointed to learn we were finished.

It was time to call the mortuary – but the family hadn't chosen one. The daughter and I walked to the nursing station and one of the nurses suggested one nearby when she saw us fumbling with a phone book (yes, this death visit happened that long ago) and we called and then I was done for the night.

I had another patient who appeared to be on the opposite end of the economic scale from that family: she seemed rich, judging by her neighborhood, her clothes, and her antique furniture. She was old and frail, and she lived alone in a large and silent apartment with high ceilings and hardwood floors that echoed as she made her way cautiously across the room. It was dark, probably because she had no need to turn the lights on: she was blind. Her son had bought it for her when he moved her across the country after her husband died, and he had also paid someone to arrange the furniture; an admission note warned us not to move anything, because she might trip over it if we did. I was surprised she didn't have a paid companion. Someone came in once a week to sweep the floors and do the laundry, and prepare meals and arrange them in the refrigerator so she could heat them in the microwave. I hoped her bedroom was cheerier than her living room, but I never saw it. On the several times I visited her, I felt I'd been inserted into a British movie starring a very polite woman who was willing to receive me although we had little in common. She had no interest in talking about her inner life.

We met with her son when she first came on our service. He was an imposing middle-aged man in a business suit, glancing at his watch and nearly tapping his foot with impatience while we introduced ourselves. I learned that he and his wife visited the patient on Sundays, and I think she went to his house on Thanksgiving and Christmas. I left perfunctory messages on his voicemail after my visits. He didn't return my calls.

Then her health began to decline rapidly, and I read that she was now bedridden; that she was on oxygen; that there was a paid caregiver at her side; that she was struggling, and then she was dead.

I made a routine condolence call to her son. This time he answered his phone, and asked if I could meet him at his mother's that afternoon. He was in the parking lot when I arrived, bundling an armful of her clothes into his car. When he turned and saw me, he began crying. I stepped toward him. I had little relationship with this big powerful man, but I opened my arms and he let me hold him while he stood in the parking lot and sobbed because his mother had died. I offered to perform a funeral or memorial service, but he refused. He called me several times over the next months to talk about what a wonderful mother she had been.

When a family doesn't belong to a church but they want a service after a death, I'm often asked to be the officiant, the one chosen to help a room full of sad people grapple with what's just happened. The first time this happened, I had only been working as a hospice chaplain for a few months, and the service was for a coworker's friend who had committed suicide. I said yes, finding the confidence they needed me to have, and then listened while the dead man's powerful friends created a ceremony. I've been using the format they devised ever since, adding and subtracting music and readings and whatever else might help.

I usually wear a simple Zen priest's work robe that identifies me as clergy. I set up an altar with a candle, some flowers, and a picture of the person who's died. I greet the assembly, introduce myself, and explain what we're going to do. I invite people to settle for a moment, step back and wait until the room is completely silent, and then ring my bell. I usually open with a poem. I invite one person to come up and tell us about the person who died. When they're done, I invite anyone else to offer a memory. And I close with a blessing. I have several options in the binder I carry, ranging from completely secular to very religious. And that's it. It's simple, it's satisfactory, and it doesn't require me to offer idle speculation about the afterlife.

I've come to see that the first and biggest step in grief is to understand that the person has died, and a good funeral can help. I appreciate graveside services, the coffin, the hole in the ground with astroturf draped around it, the friends and family standing alongside, and the workers waiting at a distance to shovel the dirt in. When families say they want a celebration of life immediately after a death, I suggest they wait a few months for grief to settle if what they want is balloons and a party in the back yard. I believe a funeral is meant to create a safe space for us to come together and be sad over a loss, not to have a party. But I've performed funerals, memorial services, and celebrations of life in all sorts of places.

I've been asked to perform Buddhist services for people born in Japan who never joined a temple in America, but whose families want to be sure their loved one makes it to the other shore after death. For these I bring incense and chant in Japanese. I've done funerals where awkward-looking young men in stiff uniforms pressed the button on a CD player to play taps as they presented the widow with a folded flag. I once arrived to perform a memorial service in a restaurant and, instead of being shown to the private room I expected, I read my prayers and blessings for four people at a table in a noisy dining room while the waitress waited to take our orders.

Once I was asked to officiate at a double funeral. The patient was an old lady who lived in a facility for people with dementia. Her daughter visited often, and had a reputation among the staff for being dramatic and demanding. The manager whispered something about drinking being involved. She and I occasionally crossed paths, and she told me how much she loved her mother and didn't want her to die. After the death, we talked, and she asked me to per-form a memorial service in a restaurant that she and her mother had loved. I agreed, and a date was set. Shortly after that, I received a second phone call, this one from the patient's granddaughter. She was crying when she told me that her mother had been found dead, felled by her grief. She asked me to perform a service for our patient and her daughter together. We kept the date and place her mother and I had agreed on.

When I arrived that day, I saw the place the two women had loved wasn't really a restaurant. We were in a bar, in a side room with a small table at one end that held a dis-play of flowers and two urns of ashes. The grand-daughter was sitting next to it and sobbing. The cash register was in the other room through an open archway, so we heard its ca-ching every time it rang up a sale. Business was brisk. The room was crowded. A few people found chairs to perch on, but most were standing, holding little plates of food in one hand and drinks in the other. When everyone seemed to be there, I rang my bell and spoke into a micro-phone, introduced myself and started my poem. Some people kept eating and drinking, nodding gravely while they listened to what was being said. The patient's grand-daughter, the young woman who had lost both her mother and her grandmother, was devastated and I was glad to see a clutch of women gathered around her when the ceremony was over. I wasn't sure our party-with-prayer had worked, but I did my best.

Of course I have opinions. It helps to remember that I'm there to embody a role, not to tell people what I think they're doing wrong. People often don't seem to know how they're supposed to behave around death, so I've had to learn how to keep my opinions to myself, quiet my mind and put a neutral expression on my face, while I witness and play my part.

Still, the opinions are there, and they extend to the local mortuaries. Hospice workers aren't supposed to recommend a mortuary, a care home, or an agency. I guess this is to avoid the appearance of graft or maybe my bosses are afraid something will go wrong and we'll be blamed. But I've seen shocking things happen when a guy in a suit arrives to take a body away, and I've been amazed by how clueless and rude some of the people who work in funeral parlors are. I don't tell my family members these stories when they ask for help, but I do give them the names of the places I like. I tell them I look for respect, for people who are kind, and for a good price.

The majority of our families choose cremation, and it happens that I have an unusual amount of experience with this, since in my tradition we perform a wonderful ceremony with the body at the crematorium. The corpse is present in a cardboard coffin, and we usually remove the lid so we can see the face of the one we love already altered by death. We perform a ritual to say goodbye and then chant while we watch the body go into the flames. It's convincing.

We need to know the person is gone before real grief can begin. People will say they don't want to see someone who's dying or dead "because I want to remember her the way she was," and they stand a good chance of being the ones who have trouble with grief, the ones who will say months later "I still can't believe she's dead" and "I keep waiting for her to call me on the phone." I encourage people to take their time when death occurs, to let the emotions settle, to open a window and let the spirit fly out, to come together and bathe the body to prepare it for what's to come. If someone is in a facility, California law says that the corpse has to be removed within four hours, but a body can remain at home for as long as the survivors need it to.

Early in my chaplaincy, I had a wife who wanted to keep her husband home for several days after he died. I was able to explain that the body should be in a cool room, and she should put dry ice under the kidneys to slow its decay. She took care of it. I visited about a day after he died, and it was a beautiful scene. He was lying on a bed in a dim room. There was a large flower arrangement on a side table. He was dressed in a shirt and tie and there was a silk cloth over the lower part of his body. He was peaceful. On the other side of the door, friends were visiting with the widow, having a cup of tea and a snack, moving through the couple's house, telling stories and offering comfort. She called the undertakers after two days and they removed him.

One family asked me to witness their mother's cremation. They wanted to be sure the mortuary had the right body, and they couldn't bear to do it themselves. I drove alone to the crematorium where the boss proudly showed me the huge refrigerator where bodies stay while the wheels of bureaucracy take care of business, and then he wheeled the large cardboard box out, took off the lid and pulled the plastic from the patient's face, and left me alone with her. I talked to her, told her that her children were full of sorrow but I was sure they'd be all right because they were supporting each other in their grief. I told her she looked great. I put the lid back on and went and found the mortician, and together we watched the coffin roll into the fire. He let me push the button that started it.

When people are grieving they naturally turn to the hospice workers for guidance. That's what we're there for. But then there are cases where the family has different ideas. There was a patient who had refused to see me, but after she died her husband asked if I could visit. They lived in a poor part of town, and their little apartment was still stuffed with medical supplies and equipment I hoped he wouldn't need any time soon. He told me he was a blues singer and she played piano, but they'd had to take other jobs to get by. He said he wanted me to help with the funeral. I explained my usual format to him and he agreed that it sounded perfect. In the event, 12 of us gathered in a run down funeral parlor I hadn't been to before. The patient was in an open casket, and as I stood at his side to see her for the first time, I noticed there were signs of wear and tear on the white satin lining. I guessed this must be a display casket people could rent for funerals, and then bury the body in something simpler. This was all new to me.

I prepared my papers and bell at the podium, and then sat in the front pew, ready to open at the signal. Then the widower stood up at the microphone, summoned a drummer, a guitar player, and a keyboard man from the assembly, and began singing. The funeral was beginning without me. He started with "Amazing Grace," of course, but before you knew it the joint was jumping to a great version of "Caledonia." For two hours he called songs and musicians. Guitarists, keyboard players and vocalists rotated through. A fabulous guy arrived in a shiny suit with a receding hairline who hadn't given up his pompadour. He was the harmonica player. There was a short plump saxophone player who kept smiling at me. Everyone in the place had gray hair, and everyone in the place had been learning their instrument for a long time. When the spirit moved him, the widower called me up and I talked about love and read a Maya Angelou poem. The chaplain was just another member of the band. It was one of my favorite funerals ever.

In all of these cases, I was making up a ritual as I went. Goodness knows, I was trained strictly and thoroughly in ritual in my years at Zen Center. I can wear three layers of voluminous Japanese robes without tripping over them, and I can – well, I could – do 27 full bows, all the way from standing to touching my forehead to the ground, during morning service. I can ring a bell at exactly the right time and I can lead a chant in Japanese with confidence. The part of this that has been useful to me in my life as a chaplain is learning to act with authority. And there is no story where this was more useful than the story of the patient who needed an exorcism. I doubt many priests, let alone chaplains, have the opportunity to perform an exorcism. I did, once -- and the best thing was, it worked.

One of our social workers called to ask for help with a young Japanese woman. She told me the doctors were working on controlling the pain that came with the patient's cancer, but the patient said spirits had taken over her mind. That's where she thought I might be able to help. I was glad she trusted me, and hurried to her office so we could talk about the case.

She explained that sometimes the patient was silent, head tilted, listening as the spirits spoke to her, and other times she shouted in Japanese, apparently becoming the spirits and broadcasting them to the world. She was living at home with her mother, who had come from Japan to take care of her. The spirits weren't evil. The problem was, their talking kept her awake all night. She and her mother were both exhausted.

I said of course I'd do it – in fact, I had time to see the patient that very afternoon. I didn't mention that, although

I'd been thoroughly trained as a Zen priest, exorcism had never come up. I felt sure I'd performed enough ceremonies that I could create one for the patient that would be convincing. We speculated about the cause of the phenomenon of the spirits, but what we thought in the safety of our office and what I saw when I entered the patient's house were completely different.

I heard the patient before I saw her. She was in a room at the end of the hallway, howling and leaning forward on a walker, the top of her head pressed against the wall. I hurried to her, dropped my bag in a chair, and sat on the floor so my face was close to hers. I could see her arms quiver from the stress of holding up her body. Her face, when she turned it toward mine, was surprising: I hadn't expected her to be so young and pretty.

I told her I was a priest, and that the social worker had sent me to help.

She answered, "They want to go to heaven."

From this moment on, we were in her reality – and it was a relief to hear the spirits were ready to go.

Now all I had to do was provide a pathway for them.

I asked her whether she'd like to sit down. She agreed, and her mother and I helped her lower her body into a white plastic chair. I never learned why she had been standing in that tortured way.

She sat on one side of a large kitchen table; her cell phone, wallet, pill bottles, note pads, Japanese newspapers and other clutter were spread out before her. Her mother stood facing her, by the stove: she was small, anxious, and a long way from home.

I cleared off a couple of square feet on the short side of the table and said it would be our altar. I set out my ritual items: two fancy incense bowls; a candle; a figure of Manjushri poised to cut through all delusions with his sword, and a small figure of Quan Yin, the bodhisattva of compassion.

I asked for flowers, and her mother rushed to the other room and brought back a vase with camellias and pine boughs. Realizing I'd left my bell in the car, I asked if they had one; they did not, and I decided to go ahead without it. What mattered now was to maintain momentum.

My *rakusu* is the garment that shows I've taken priestly vows; I put it on my head and said, as I have done hundreds of times when entering a sacred space, *Great robe of liberation / Field far beyond form and emptiness / Wearing the Tatagatha's teaching, / Saving all beings* and I began.

I explained I was going to perform a Buddhist ritual to help the spirits that were inhabiting the patient go to heaven. I asked the patient and her mother to do three bows to the altar with me. Lighting a stick of incense, I pressed it against my forehead and the foreheads of the Manjushri and Quan Yin statues, and placed it upright in the first incense bowl. Then I began chanting and putting pinches of chip incense on the red-hot charcoal in the second bowl to create clouds of smoke. The room began to smell wonderful. My voice filled the space as I began to chant to Quan Yin, *Kanzeon / namu butsu / yo butsu u in / yo butsu u en / buppo so en / jo raku ga jo / cho nen kanzeon / bo nen kanzeon / nen nen ju shin ki / nen nen fu ri shin.* The chant is simple and can be repeated endlessly, and the compassion of Quan Yin was what we needed.

I chanted, waiting to see what would happen, when suddenly the patient cried out, rose from her chair, and stepped toward me, shaking her head violently and yelling "No! No! No!"

She clutched my upper arms. I leaned forward and grabbed her above the waist to keep her from falling. I kept chanting. She kept shaking her head. Her short black hair, inches from my face, smelled clean and fresh. I somehow held her body with one arm so I could use the other to put more incense on the charcoal. The smoke billowed in the room and I began to speak to the spirit, loudly, firmly, invoking all of the authority I had in me:

"You hungry ghost, haunting ladies on this plane, it's time for you to be released. Follow the smoke to heaven! With this ceremony you can let go and your wish will come true! The time is now!"

She continued to shake her head. She cried out that he couldn't let go.

I was still bent forward, holding her.

"Don't be afraid!" I called. "You have courage! You know courage! Use that courage now to let go of this woman, let go and go to heaven at last!"

Now, I can't say how long this went on. Then, it seemed timeless, the two (or three) of us locked in this quasi-embrace, incense smoke and my voice filling the kitchen, her mother nearby, watching us, crying and wringing her hands.

My back hurt from supporting the patient, but I continued until she calmed; then I signaled to the mother to move the chair forward so I could ease her into it. I pressed my back against the kitchen wall to ease the pain and continued the chant to Quan Yin in a softer voice.

Finally the young woman looked up at me and smiled. She nodded her head.

"Is he gone?"

"Yes."

And then she said, "But the others are still here."

I hadn't known that there were others.

I stepped back in front of the altar, threw more incense on the charcoal, resumed the chant in a louder voice, and then called out to the lesser spirits that they could follow the boss's example and go to heaven. I told them this was their chance. Much more quickly this time, she nodded her head and said they were gone. I finished the chant, offered a dedication of gratitude, and the three of us did three bows to close the ceremony. I passed the figure of Quan

Yin through the remaining incense smoke and gave it to her.

That was an hour's work. I was exhausted.

The magic I'd brought that day resided in my vow as a priest, my beautiful Japanese ritual implements, and my willingness to believe the young woman's description of her reality. On that day, we trusted each other, and it worked. I phoned the social worker from my car to report on our success, and she and I cried together.

I spoke to the patient on the phone the next day. The spirits were gone, and she and her mother been able to sleep through the night.

The doctors admitted her to the hospital that day and, to my relief, she was referred to the medical ward for pain control, not to the psych ward for the spirits that had inhabited her.

She died at home two weeks later. The spirits never returned.

Sometimes I feel jealous of my Christian coworkers who are given prayers to recite and ceremonies to perform. It looks easy. I love watching a Catholic priest arrive, don a strip of sacred cloth, inscribe an ancient symbol in the air, and read words of comfort that are designed to send a dying person to heaven. But it's not my way. Zen has taught me the value of spontaneity, of trusting my training and my sincerity to bring forth words that will offer confidence and comfort when they're needed, and that's the ritual I bring with me during and after a death.

What Good is Life

Once in a moment of frustration, I asked my Zen teacher "What good is Zen?" Without hesitation he responded "What good is life?"

Well, that's the question.

I heard in AA that the antidote to pain was to help others, and that's a good start. Around the same time, all those decades ago, I heard an Episcopal priest say we should follow Jesus' teaching and love one another. That seemed right, but I wanted to raise my hand and ask him how to do it.

It was my longing to learn the answer to that question that drove me to the radical step of leaving my conventional life and moving to a Zen monastery when I was in my late 50s, and that same yearning is what drove me to train as a chaplain when I was in my mid-60s. I wanted to live a good life. I wanted to learn how to love and be loved.

I recently visited a young woman who was dying of cancer. She was gaunt and spoke little while her husband carried the rage and sorrow for both of them. Together they'd been through the medical system, and he complained of doctors who seemed more interested in their computers than in her. "They never listened," he said.

I listened. I let in the hopelessness of the situation, the powerlessness of everyone in the room as the young woman's body continued its march toward death. I locked eyes with her and I listened to him.

And then I talked. I described hospice, how our clients qualify and what we do. I described the likely trajectory of her life, the increasing weakness and loss of appetite, then becoming bedridden, and then "the chances are good that one day you'll fall asleep and not wake up." I assured her that our people are good at pain control. When I saw that I was tiring her, I said it was time to leave. She thanked me for coming and, her voice suddenly strong, asked me to come again soon.

Why, I wondered when I left. What help had I been, really, in this tragic situation? Which of the informational threads I'd picked up and offered had been of help to her? Later, I thought, what I did was, I met her gaze. I wasn't afraid of her ravaged face and her silence. She was a devout Catholic and here I was looking not like another medical professional but like a physical reminder of the spiritual side of life, and I didn't need to do or say anything for that to be comforting. She said she believed that each of us has a destiny, and this was hers. I could smile and nod and accept that, even though it's the polar opposite of my belief. There was connection.

And of all the words I said, it was the words about love that mattered: the love I saw in the room between the patient, her husband, and the friend who was staying with them. The love that I offered as the only possible response to their – and our – hopeless situation.

She died before I could see her again.

Not long ago, I too was diagnosed with cancer.

I had noticed a bump on my upper arm that didn't go away. When I was seeing my dermatologist for something else, I asked her to take a look. She said to come back in a month if it was still there; when I did, she took a biopsy. Two weeks later, she called and said it was lymphoma. I bent toward the desk and pulled a pad over to write the word down. I'd need to look at it again so I could absorb this news. I also wrote down the word "radiation."

The doctor's call came just as I was leaving to go and lead my weekly meditation group. It was useful to be forced to sit still in silence just then. I could feel the fear in my body, and greet it, as my Zen teacher had taught, without turning away. By the end of that period of meditation, I understood that whatever happened, it would be fine. This is my understanding of Zen: whatever happens is fine.

The hospital put me through tests and probes for two weeks before I met with my new oncologist. I spent too much time online - but of course I did - and learned that cutaneous B-cell lymphoma is slow growing, and still I was consumed by anxiety. I thought I saw somewhere that the five year survival rate was 60% which meant I had a 40% chance of dying from this little red bump. I had trouble eating and sleeping, and couldn't work. I called a few friends and told them what was going on, and they were eager to help.

I'll admit there was some relief mixed in with the fear and anxiety. Working in hospice and seeing hundreds of deaths, I wonder how mine will be, and there are many diseases that frighten me more than cancer. So now I had a feeling of "Ah, so it's you! So this is your name!" I was old enough to say I wasn't too young to die. I was also young enough that I had good years in front of me if this truly was nothing.

I had two oncologists. I liked the first one. She said a cancer like this is just a matter of the law of averages: as we age, the chances increase that one or two of our cells will go crazy and that's how we end up in her office. She said the cancer was slow growing and we'd caught it early. It hadn't spread. My five year survival rate, at least from this lymphoma, was 100%. She let me interrupt and ask my questions. She was reassuring.

The other oncologist was the one who guided my daily radiation sessions at the cancer center. I was quivering with anxiety and she belittled me, scorned my emotions, and suggested I might need therapy or Prozac. She never asked whether my anxiety was a problem for me, but it sure was a problem for her.

Radiation made me so tired. I spent long afternoons lying on the couch watching non-challenging television. Friends brought me soup and flowers. I needed distraction so I fell in love with a longtime friend who had showed up to help. He gave my mind a place to land when I felt lonely during the day or anxiety woke me in the night.

I grasped for control of my life as I free-floated through the unknown. I've talked to scores of hospice patients about this, as they tell me what they want to happen, that they think they should live for a certain amount of time and die in a certain way, and yet it was hard for me to remember that I couldn't control my cancer, and then I had to remember over and over. I wished there was someone who could tell me what was going on, help me understand my reaction to radiation and let me know what to expect. I promised myself to try to be that person for my patients when I returned to work.

One morning when the radiation sickness was strongest, I stood in the shower and laughed because I thought I had found the answer and then watched it escape my grasp. It was like being on LSD. Driving to the cancer center that day, I saw the thoughts form again, and I pulled over and scribbled them down: what you're looking for doesn't come from the outside. It doesn't lie in having enough friends, as I thought when I didn't have any; or even in being helpful for a living, as I thought when I was first learning how to be a priest/chaplain. Being connected

-- having friends and being helpful -- is a way of life, not a cure for it. Looking for meaning, which is what this is really about, is standing in the river and crying because I'm thirsty.

Now I'm changed, and the post-lymphoma phase centers on meeting this new formulation of me. All of the elements in my life are still there, but they're each in a new place, in a new relationship to each other, and I have to learn the territory all over again. What I've lost seems to be my sense of my own immortality. Perhaps what I've gained is an end to the question my teacher threw back at me ten years ago when I asked "What good is Zen?" and he asked "What good is life?"

A basic teaching in Buddhism is of groundlessness. Everything is always changing, so there's no firm place to stand. This is one of those teachings that's easier to read about than to live. I don't forget that the phone can ring and someone can say a word like "cancer" and life will change. The hospice company you loved can be mismanaged and most of your friends can be laid off or quit, as happened at mine that year. Your lover can walk out the door at 2 am and never return, and that happened too. This is groundlessness, and the trick is not to get lost in yearning for the way things used to be or dreaming about creating a new nest to settle into, but to live with life as it is.

It's quite a trick.

Years ago I was visiting a woman who had been in a coma for days. She suddenly sat up and looked me in the eye and said "Dying is hard work." I believed her. Living is hard work, too. And so is love.

I think back to those first lessons I learned when I was training in the hospital: represent the spiritual side of life in the way you look and act; don't turn away when it's hard and you're flying alone and blind; trust your instinct and step forward to help; reach into the connection that's already there and let it manifest in the room. Be willing to be vulnerable. Be kind.

I don't talk much about God in my work any more, but I talk about love. In a world of turmoil in which many of us are wondering what we should do, I urge patients and friends alike: love more. The world needs more love, let's create it, I say, and we smile together, as I did with the gaunt young woman with cancer who died so rapidly.

Now here I am, all of me, turning again to my vow – the promises I've made times beyond numbering since I first ordained as a Zen Buddhist –

Beings are numberless, I vow to save them
Delusions are inexhaustible, I vow to end them
Dharma gates are boundless, I vow to enter them
Buddha's way is unsurpassable, I vow to become it

– the promises that are obviously impossible to attain and yet remain alive in every breath to support me through the pleasure and the pain of being human, of seeing fear and choosing love.

Further Reading

Here are some books about death and dying by Buddhist teachers that I like and recommend

The Five Invitations: Discovering What Death Can Teach Us About Living Fully by Frank Ostaseski

The Art of Dying Well: A Practical Guide to a Good End of Life, and *Knocking on Heaven's Door* by Katy Butler

Being with Dying: Cultivating Compassion and Fearlessness in the Presence of Death and *Standing at the Edge: Finding Freedom where Fear and Courage Meet* by Joan Halifax

Wholehearted: Slow Down, Help Out, Wake Up by Koshin Paley Ellison and *Awake at the Bedside* edited by Koshin Paley Ellison and Matt Weingast

A Beginner's Guide to the End: Practical Advice for Living Life and Facing Death by BJ Miller and Shoshanna Berger

Advice for Future Corpses (and Those Who Love Them): A Practical Perspective on Death and Dying by Sallie Tisdale

And allow me to mention my previous book:
Entering the Monastery by Renshin Bunce

202

When I finished *Entering the Monastery* in 2017, I self-published it as an offering to my friends. When I was writing *Love and Fear*, I thought it would have wider appeal than that story of my life at San Francisco Zen Center, and hoped to get it published commercially. The several agents who I submitted it to disagreed, so I'm self-publishing this one too.

The Well has been my online home for several decades, and friends there helped me with the technical problems that arose in formatting the Word doc that gets uploaded to create the book. I designed the cover using one of my own photos, and that too was prepared for uploading by a friend on The Well.

I've used the picture Shundo David Haye took of me for the author photo on the back cover.

The book isn't perfect, but it is offered with a sincere heart. Thank you for reading it.

Made in the USA
Las Vegas, NV
19 November 2020